Ocular Immunology in Health and Disease

Ocular Immunology in Health and Disease

Steven B. Koevary, Ph.D.

Associate Professor of Immunology, Ocular Research Center, New England College of Optometry, Boston; Adjunct Associate Professor of Cell Biology, University of Massachusetts Medical School, Worcester

BUTTERWORTH
HEINEMANN

Boston   Oxford   Auckland   Johannesburg   Melbourne   New Delhi

Inset on front cover reprinted with permission from PG McMenamin, J Crewe. Endotoxin-induced uveitis: kinetics and phenotype of the inflammatory cell infiltrate and the response of the resident tissue macrophages and dendritic cells in the iris and ciliary body. Invest Ophthalmol Vis Sci 1995;36(18):front cover. Copyright 1995. Association for Research in Vision and Ophthalmology.

Library of Congress Cataloging-in-Publication Data
Koevary, Steven B.
    Ocular immunology in health and disease / Steven B. Koevary.
        p.   cm.
    Includes bibliographical references and index.
    ISBN 0-7506-9900-0
    1. Eye--Immunology. 2. Eye--Diseases--Immunological aspects.
    I. Title.
        [DNLM: 1. Eye--immunology. 2. Eye Diseases--immunology. WW 140
    K78o 1999]
    RE68.K64 1999
    617.7'1--dc21
    DNLM/DLC
    for Library of Congress   98-46553
                                                                         CIP

British Library Cataloguing-in-Publication Data
A catalogue record for this book is available from the British Library.

The publisher offers special discounts on bulk orders of this book.
For information, please contact:

Manager of Special Sales
Butterworth–Heinemann
225 Wildwood Avenue
Woburn, MA 01801-2041
Tel: 781-904-2500
Fax: 781-904-2620

For information on all Butterworth–Heinemann publications available,
contact our World Wide Web home page at: http://www.bh.com

10 9 8 7 6 5 4 3 2 1

Printed in the United States of America

To my wife, Shira, and my children,
Elayna, Benjamin, and Yael

In memoriam: Raphael Persky

Contents

Preface

Immune processes play an important role in combating ocular infection and preventing ocular tumors. Elements of the immune system mediate ocular allergy as well as ocular and systemic autoimmunity, the latter of which may indirectly affect the eye. Finally, immune processes play a role in the rejection of foreign grafts such as corneal allografts.

This book elucidates the role of the immune system in mediating these effects in a way that will benefit not only optometry and ophthalmology students but also clinicians who wish to stay current in this field. The primary objectives are to give an accurate and current overview of immune system function, especially as it relates to systemic and ocular disease, and to elaborate on the role of immune effector mechanisms in specific ocular conditions.

The book begins with an overview of the immune system and proceeds to concentrate on the unique aspects of ocular immunology, including a discussion of specific ocular conditions in which immune cells and factors play an important part, such as allergy and autoimmunity. The book ends with a consideration of the immune system's role in ocular tumor elimination and corneal transplantation.

STEVEN B. KOEVARY

Acknowledgments

I wish to acknowledge the organizational and editorial assistance of Kristin Robinson, a research technician in my laboratory, and the editorial assistance of Jana Friedman and Karen Oberheim of Butterworth–Heinemann and Kim Langford of Silverchair Science + Communications.

Ocular Immunology in Health and Disease

CHAPTER 1

Overview of the Human Immune System

The above results show that cell fusion techniques are a powerful tool to produce a specific antibody directed against a predetermined antigen. It is further demonstrated that it is possible to isolate hybrid lines producing different antibodies directed against the same antigen and carrying different effector functions.

Such cultures could be valuable for medical and industrial use.*

Although empirical observations about immunity date back to ancient times, it was the exposition of the germ theory in the late nineteenth century that represents the birth of immunologic science. This theory was supported by the experiments of such investigators as Robert Koch and Louis Pasteur. The theory held that infectious agents did not arise by spontaneous generation but that they could reproduce and were specific for different disease entities. Since that time, there have been great strides made in our understanding of how the immune system works to protect us from infectious microbes such as bacteria, viruses, fungi, and parasites, as well as from the unfettered growth of body cells that have become neoplastic.

This chapter is devoted to a review of immune system function. Where appropriate, references are made to the ocular immune response though this topic is discussed in more specific detail in Chapter 3. First, the general organization of the immune system is discussed and its component cells, tissues, and factors are described. An analysis of how an immune response is generated against specific pathogens follows. The nature of hypersensitivity reactions, transplantation, tumor immunology, and autoimmunity is then discussed, and the chapter ends with a discussion of congenital and acquired immunodeficiencies, including acquired immunodeficiency syndrome (AIDS).

---

*From the landmark paper by Nobel Prize–winning scientists Georges Kohler and Cesar Milstein that launched the monoclonal antibody field (G Kohler, C Milstein. Continuous cultures of fused cells secreting antibody of predefined specificity. Nature 1975;256:495–497).

TABLE 1.1
Barrier Defenses of the Innate, or Nonadaptive, Immune System

Physical Barriers	*Biochemical Barriers*
Skin	Mucous glycoproteins
Conjunctiva	Acid in stomach
Gastrointestinal tract mucous membranes	Lactic acid in female reproductive tract
	Lysozyme in tears and other fluids
Respiratory tract mucous membranes	Lactoferrin in tears and other fluids
Cilia lining respiratory tract	Beta-lysin in tears and other fluids
Genitourinary tract mucous membranes	C-reactive protein in serum
	Complement proteins in serum
	Sebaceous gland secretions

Organization of the Immune System

The immune system evolved as a means of protecting the body from pathogenic organisms including viruses, bacteria, fungi, and protozoan and multicellular parasites, as well as from cancerous cell growth. To a certain extent, protection from some viruses goes hand in hand with the prevention of tumor growth because some viruses are known to induce neoplastic transformation in cells.

The immune system consists of two functional divisions that act together to prevent infection: (1) an innate, natural, or nonadaptive immunity, and (2) an adaptive, or specific, immunity.

Innate or Natural Immunity

The innate response is characterized by a limited capacity to distinguish between pathogens, a stereotypic response to these organisms, and an absence of memory. This latter point refers to the fact that the innate immune response to a particular agent is not enhanced by previous exposure to it. Constituents of the innate response include physical and chemical barriers (Table 1.1), blood proteins, and inflammatory cells.

Physical and Chemical Barriers

The physical barriers include the skin; conjunctiva; and mucous membranes surrounding the respiratory, gastrointestinal, urinary, and reproductive tracts. It is important to remember that for an infectious agent to gain entry into the body, an epithelial barrier must be breached. As a further innate protection of these epithelial barriers, they are bathed in protective mucus or a serous secretion containing antimicrobial compounds. For example, lysozyme, lactoferrin, beta-lysin, and various complement proteins are found in the tear film overlying the conjunctival and corneal epithelia. Similar constituents are found in the fluid overlying the respiratory and gastrointestinal mucosa. Lactic acid produced by bacteria in the female reproductive tract and acid produced in the stomach protect these regions from bacterial growth.

Acute Phase Proteins

In addition to the factors mentioned above, a host of serum proteins called *acute phase proteins* are secreted primarily by the liver and increase rapidly in concentration in response to infection. These include C-reactive protein (CRP), type I interferon (IFN), and the complement proteins. CRP binds to molecular groups on a wide variety of bacteria and fungi and, by so doing, facilitates their uptake by phagocytic cells. In this context, CRP is said to act as an opsonin in a process of facilitated phagocytosis called *opsonization*. Certain complement proteins can also act as opsonins, as can antibodies (which are elements of the adaptive immune response). Interestingly, high levels of CRP in the blood were shown to correlate with increased risk of heart attack, supporting a role for vascular inflammation in plaque formation.[1]

Type I IFN consists collectively of IFN-α, secreted primarily by mononuclear phagocytes, and IFN-β, secreted by fibroblasts. These factors play an important role in limiting the spread of viral infection. Specifically, they accomplish this by inducing enzymes, such as 2′,5′-oligoadenylate synthetase, that interfere with the replication of viral RNA and DNA. Furthermore, they increase major histocompatibility complex (MHC) expression on cells, facilitating their destruction by cytotoxic T lymphocytes, as explained later. In destroying virally infected cells, the immune system eliminates the viral factories that are the source for systemic viral dissemination. Type I IFN also increases the activity of natural killer (NK) cells; these cells play a surveillance role in innate immunity by seeking out virally infected cells and killing them in less time than it would take cytotoxic T cells.

Complement comprises a series of effector and regulatory serum proteins that play a role in the innate, as well as adaptive, immune responses. These proteins circulate in the blood and are present in extracellular tissues. Complement proteins are known to mediate five effector functions. As listed below, the first three are elements of innate immunity and the last two are elements of the adaptive response:

1. Osmotic lysis of bacteria and body cells by polymerization into a pore structure;
2. Opsonization of microorganisms facilitating their phagocytosis by macrophages and neutrophils;
3. Chemotactic attraction of leukocytes to a site of infection;
4. Solubilization of immune complexes thus preventing them from inducing a hypersensitivity reaction (discussed later in the chapter); and
5. Promoting the localization of antigens (antigens are molecules that can be specifically recognized by elements of adaptive immunity and

TABLE 1.2
Functions of Complement Proteins

Osmotic lysis of bacteria
Opsonization of microorganisms
Chemotaxis
Solubilization of immune complexes
Localization of antigen to B cell nodules

---

represent fragments of foreign molecules such as viral peptides) to antibody-producing B lymphocytes and antigen-presenting cells (APCs) (discussed later in this chapter).

A summary of the functions of complement proteins appears in Table 1.2.

There are two main pathways of complement activation—the classical and the alternative—that converge at various points in an enzymatic cascade. The classical pathway is initiated as part of the adaptive immune response by the binding of antigen-bound antibodies to complement protein C1; this binding is referred to as *complement fixation*. The corneal limbus has high concentrations of C1, making it a particularly susceptible region for classical pathway activation. The alternative pathway is activated in the absence of antibody and as such is involved in innate immunity. Normally small amounts of the complement protein C3 deposit on body cells. This binding does not result in the activation of the enzymatic cascade because of the action of regulatory proteins produced by these cells. However, should microorganisms be present, they too would be coated by C3; activation would then occur because these foreign invaders fail to generate regulator proteins that inhibit the cascade. Other complement proteins involved in the alternative pathway include factors B and D.

In the course of complement activation by the above pathways, different proteins are generated. These proteins have chemotactic functions (C3a and C5a), act as opsonins (C3b and C4b), cooperate to form the cytolytic membrane attack complex (C5–C9), solubilize immune complexes (C3), and promote B cell responses (iC3b and C3dg). When complement proteins are absent for congenital reasons, the chief consequences are disseminated bacterial infections and vascular inflammation resulting from immune complex deposition.

Regulatory factors play an important role in complement activation, as alluded to earlier. Many of these factors are present in the serum and fibroblasts, as well as on blood, endothelial, and epithelial cells. One eye-related factor worth mentioning is decay-accelerating factor (DAF). It is the inability of microorganisms to express DAF, together with another regulatory factor called *membrane cofactor protein* (MCP), which accounts for the preferential activation of the alternative pathway by foreign invaders. DAF acts by dissociating the enzyme C3 convertase, which cleaves C3 to generate C3b and is necessary for the continuation of the cascade. It is found in closed-eye tears and plays a role in the prevention of complement-mediated damage in that tissue environment.

Inflammatory Cells

Inflammatory cells such as macrophages and polymorphonuclear neu- trophils play an important role in innate immunity by phagocytosing a wide variety of foreign microorganisms and eliminating them. Both macrophages and neutrophils have antibody and complement receptors and thus play a role in opsonization, and both migrate and accumulate at sites of comple- ment activation in response to chemotactic agents. The specific process by which circulating blood cells insinuate themselves between neighboring endothelial cells to access the underlying tissues is referred to as *diapedesis*.

Neutrophils belong to the group of blood cells termed *granulocytes*, together with eosinophils and basophils, because they possess specific granules that participate in the immune response. The specific granules in neutrophils contain lysozyme and lactoferrin. Eosinophil-specific granules contain major basic protein (MBP), eosinophil peroxidase (EPO), eosinophil cationic protein (ECP), and eosinophil-derived neurotoxin (EDN). Although eosinophils can be phagocytic, their primary role is in the immune response to parasites and in certain types of allergic reactions. Basophil- specific granules contain heparin and leukotrienes, which, when released, mediate systemic anaphylaxis.

Adaptive or Specific Immunity

The characteristics of adaptive immunity are nearly the opposite of those described for innate immunity. Adaptive immunity is characterized by the ability to distinguish between pathogenic organisms (i.e., specificity), and by the enhanced intensity of responsiveness on secondary exposure to a pathogen (i.e., memory). Furthermore, though the temporal dynamics of the innate response are rapid, specific immunity requires more time to become fully active (Figure 1.1). Constituents of specific immunity include T and B lymphocytes, APCs, and plasma cells. APCs are given different names depending on their location; examples include the dendritic cells in lymph nodes and Langerhans' cells in the skin and eye.

Cellular and Humoral Immune Responses

Specific immunity has two major subdivisions: the cellular and humoral immune responses. The cellular immune response, mediated by T cells and APCs, plays an important role in the elimination of intracellular infec- tion by viruses and fungi, in the elimination of cancer cells, and in the destruction of foreign tissue grafts. T cells can be subdivided into helper T cells, which express the surface marker CD4 and cytotoxic killer cells, which express CD8. T helper cells can be further subdivided into T helper

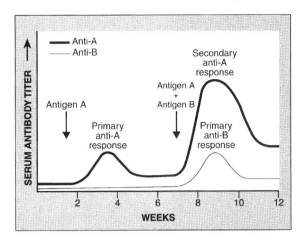

FIGURE 1.1.   Specificity and memory of the adaptive immune response. (Reprinted with permission from AK Abbas, AH Lichtman, JS Pober. Cellular and Molecular Immunology [3rd ed]. Philadelphia: Saunders, 1997;8.)

1 (Th1) cells, which secrete factors that play a role in cellular immunity and Th2 cells, which secrete factors that assist in the production of antibody by B cells in response to "T-dependent antigens," such as proteins and polymeric antigens (such as polysaccharides). Certain T cells have the capacity to downregulate immune responses and are referred to as suppressor or regulatory cells.

Humoral immunity involves the production of antibody by plasma cells, which are the differentiation end products of B lymphocyte activation. As alluded to above, T cells (and APCs) may also be involved in the production of antibody by B cells. The humoral immune response plays a particularly important role in the extracellular phases of infection. For example, antibody binding to invading microorganisms inhibits their ability to latch on to body cells and prevents them from establishing a foothold.

Phases of the Adaptive Immune Response

The adaptive immune response to an antigen is divided into three phases: (1) a cognitive, or recognition, phase; (2) an activation phase; and (3) an effector phase. The recognition phase involves the binding of antigens to specific receptors on T or B cells. Following antigen binding, a sequence of events occurs within the immune cell resulting in the transcription of new proteins, proliferation and expansion of the activated cell, and ultimately the differentiation of the activated cell and its progeny into effector cells. All these steps comprise the activation phase. In the effector phase, effector lymphocytes either directly kill foreign invaders or infected body cells or secrete low molecular factors, called *cytokines*, which are either directly involved in the destruction of pathogens or induce other cells, such as cytotoxic T lymphocytes and macrophages, to be more efficient in their elimination of these organisms. The feature of memory in the adaptive immune response is a consequence of the retention of cells in a quasi-activation state.

Two Basic Tenets of Immunology

Clonal Selection Theory

The clonal selection theory represents the synthesis of views expressed by Jerne, Talmadge, and Burnet in the 1950s and is a unified approach to the analysis of how both T and B cells respond to antigens. Contrary to a previously held view, antigens do not indiscriminately bind to the first available T or B cell and activate it. Instead this theory states that antigens only bind to and activate T and B cells which have the appropriately matching antigen-binding receptor specificity. Once bound by antigen, these selected T and B cells clonally expand and differentiate into effector immune cells. In the case of the B cell, the antigen receptor is an integral membrane-bound antibody molecule. After antigen binding, the receptor/antigen complex moves within the plane of the membrane and aggregates to one pole of the cell by a process referred to as *capping*. This is followed by the internalization of the complexes and activation of the B cell and its differentiation into a plasma cell which secretes antibody molecules with the same specificity as its parent B cell's surface antigen receptor. This theory presupposes that each T and B cell has antigen-binding receptors with only a single specificity (Figure 1.2).

For the clonal selection to be an effective mechanism of immune activation, the T and B lymphocyte pools must contain a huge repertoire of cells with different antigen-binding specificities. This is accomplished by a variety of means including the use of different genes to encode the antigen-receptor molecules, the recombination of these genes, and, in the case of B cells, somatic mutation.

Immunologic Restriction and T Cell Activation

Immunologic responses that require the activation of T cells are governed by the law of immunologic or MHC restriction. Two important types of MHC molecules, class I and class II, are encoded in a region of chromosome 6 referred to as the *HLA region*. As a general rule, all body cells express class I antigens, whereas only cells with immune function express class II. The law of immunologic restriction states that a T cell can bind to, and be activated by, an antigen only if the antigen is "presented" to it in the context of an MHC molecule. An antigen is presented to a CD4+ helper T cell while incorporated into the class II molecule of an APC. In

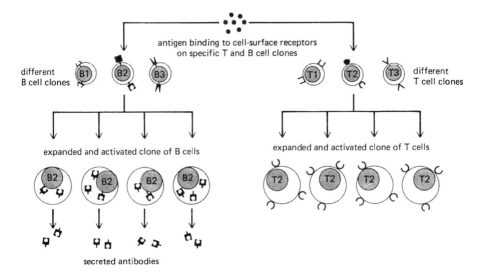

FIGURE 1.2.   The clonal selection theory. (Reprinted with permission from B Alberts, D Bray, J Lewis, et al. Molecular Biology of the Cell [2nd ed]. New York: Garland, 1989;1006.)

the case of a virally infected fibroblast, CD8+ cytotoxic T cells recognize viral antigens only when they are incorporated into the class I molecules on these cells. Thus, helper cells are said to be class II restricted, and cytotoxic cells are said to be class I restricted. In the case of both helper and cytotoxic T cells, antigen in the context of an MHC molecule binds to a specific T cell surface antigen receptor (TCR). The CD4 and CD8 molecules promote adhesion during antigen presentation and participate in the early signal transduction events that ultimately result in T cell activation. It should be mentioned that in most cases of both T and B cell antigen binding, it is only a small part, called an *antigenic determinant* or *epitope*, of the larger antigenic molecule that is required for immune activation.

Since the original elaboration of the concept of immunologic restriction, another required signal in the process of T cell activation has been discovered. This second signal is provided by what has been termed *costimulatory molecules*, which are present on the surface of APCs and bind to ligands on the T cell. The most important of these costimulatory molecules are B7-1 (CD80) and B7-2 (CD86), which bind to CD28 on the T cell. It is only when restricted antigen presentation is accompanied by the binding of costimulator molecules that T cell activation occurs (Figure 1.3). B7-1 and B7-2 also bind to CTLA-4 on T cells, but such binding was shown to inhibit rather than stimulate T cell activation. Other molecules on the surface of APCs that may act as costimulators include leukocyte function-

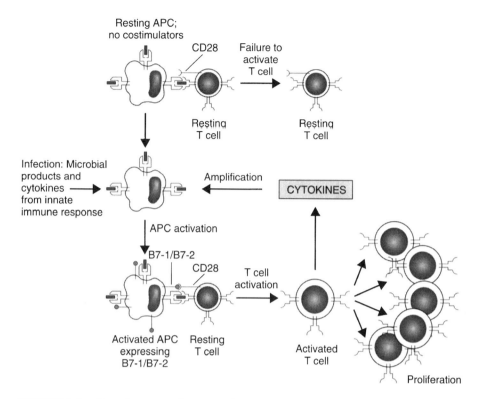

FIGURE 1.3. Requirement of costimulator molecules on antigen-presenting cells (APCs) for effective T cell activation. These costimulator molecules are upregulated by microbial products such as endotoxin and cytokines elaborated by the innate immune response. Cytokines secreted by the activated T cells can induce costimulator expression on other APCs, enabling them to serve as effective antigen presenters. (Reprinted with permission from AK Abbas, AH Lichtman, JS Pober. Cellular and Molecular Immunology [3rd ed]. Philadelphia: Saunders, 1997;156.)

associated antigen–3 (LFA-3) and intercellular adhesion molecule–1 (ICAM-1), which bind to CD2 and LFA-1, respectively, on T cells.

Organization of the Primary and Secondary Lymphoid Organs

All hematopoietic cells begin their development in the bone marrow and many complete it there, including red blood cells, granulocytes, monocytes, platelets, and B cells. T cells, on the other hand, carry out most of their differentiation in the thymus, to which they migrate from the bone marrow early in their development. Lymphocytes develop from lymphoid stem cell precursors in the bone marrow though all other blood cell elements develop from myeloid stem cell precursors. Both the thymus and bone marrow are referred to as primary lymphoid organs to characterize their primary role in lymphocyte development and differentiation. Lymphocyte activation does not occur in primary lymphoid organs but rather in the secondary lymphoid organs that include the spleen and lymph nodes. Also a part of this secondary lymphoid system are specific aggregates of lymphoid tissue found in various subepithelial locations throughout the body including the conjunctiva (conjunctiva-associated lymphoid tissue [CALT]), respiratory tract (bronchus-associated lymphoid tissue [BALT]), gastrointestinal tract (gut-associated lymphoid tissue [GALT]) of which Peyer's patches are components, the genitourinary tract, and oral cavity (tonsils). Lymphocytes in secondary lymphoid organs aggregate either diffusely or into nodules. In general, T cells are present in diffuse lymphatic tissues and B cells are located in nodular lymphatic tissue. Lymphoid nodules that respond to antigens have activated central regions called *germinal centers.*

Mature B lymphocytes that have completed their differentiation in the bone marrow migrate to the secondary lymphoid tissues where they are positioned to interact with antigens. Mature B cells express a host of cell surface molecules including immunoglobulin molecules, which serve as B cell antigen receptors, complement receptors, and immunoglobulin receptors, among others. Complement binding to B cell complement receptors is thought to play a role in augmenting the production of antibody and in promoting the binding of antigens to APCs in the germinal centers of lymphoid nodules.

Early T cell precursors that enter the thymus do so in the outer thymic cortex. These early T cells do not have a fully formed TCR or CD4 or CD8 molecules. By the time a T cell exits the cortex to enter the thymic medulla and then the circulation, it expresses its TCR and either the CD4 or CD8 molecule (though there are exceptions that are not discussed). The T cell differentiation process is facilitated by the release of thymic hormones such as thymosin and thymopoietin. Two selection processes occur in the thymus that ensure that mature T cells leaving the thymus function properly. In positive selection, T cells that have the capacity to bind to self-MHC molecules on thymic stromal cells continue their maturation, whereas those that cannot undergo apoptosis, or programmed cell death. Because T cells must recognize MHC antigens to become activated, it is clear why developing T cells that lack this ability must be eliminated. In negative selection, T cells that bind with a high affinity to self-MHC molecules presented by specialized thymic macrophages are destroyed. Because it is believed that these MHC molecules contain self-peptides in their antigen-binding groove, negative selection is postulated to be a mechanism responsible for ensuring that potentially autoreactive T cells are eliminated from the immune system. The induction of tolerance to self-antigens is an important role of the thymus, though peripheral tolerance mechanisms that induce functional immune cell inactivation or anergy have also been postulated.

Role of Antibodies and Cytokines in the Immune Response

Antibodies

Antibody or immunoglobulin molecules are secreted by plasma cells after B lymphocyte activation. They are composed of two heavy and two light chains held together by interchain disulfide bonds. The hypervariable regions in the amino terminal, or Fab, portions of the molecule contain the antigen-binding groove; these regions are hypervariable because the genes that encode their structure are multiple, undergo rearrangements, and mutate. The carboxy end of the molecule, called the *Fc region*, can bind to complement as well as to phagocytic cells by way of their Fc receptors (Figure 1.4).

There are five antibody isotypes, each containing a unique heavy-chain immunoglobulin (Ig): IgM, IgG, IgD, IgA, and IgE. IgA generally exists as a dimer, IgM as a pentamer, and all other isotypes as monomers. IgG constitutes about 75% of the total serum immunoglobulins and is the only isotype capable of crossing the placenta. It exists as four subclasses that each participate preferentially in different processes such as opsonization and complement fixation. IgA is present in only very low levels in the serum, but is present in high concentrations in body fluids such as tears, saliva, colostrum, mucus, and intestinal secretions. The role of IgA in ocular immunity is discussed in Chapter 3. IgD acts as an antigen receptor on B cells as does a special monomeric form of IgM. Because of its pentameric structure, serum IgM is the most efficient antibody involved in complement activation and also exhibits the greatest antigen-binding avidity. These features make this antibody isotype uniquely effective against invading microorganisms, and indeed, IgM is generally the first isotype released after B cell activation. The isotype of activated B cells soon switches either to IgG, IgA, or IgE, the latter of which, plays an important role in the elimination of parasites and in the allergic response.

Antibodies have various biological effects, including neutralization of antigen; activation of complement; opsonization; mediation of antibody-dependent cell-mediated cytotoxicity (ADCC) and types I, II, and III hypersensitivity reactions; and providing mucosal and neonatal immunity. Antibody-mediated antigen neutralization is the basis of vaccination protocols that protect immunized hosts against microbial toxins such as tetanus and snake venom. It is also the process by which extracellular pathogens are prevented from binding to cell surface receptors. The role of complement fixation and opsonization were discussed earlier. The process of

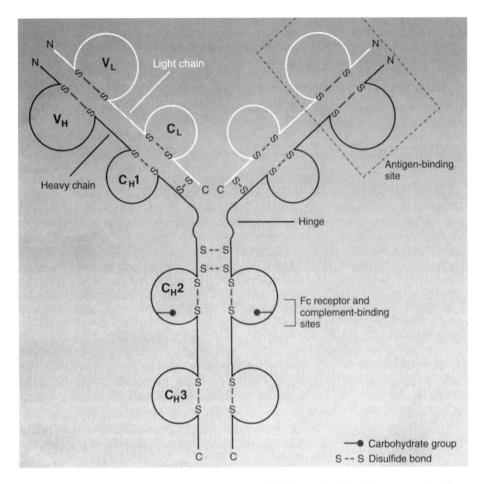

FIGURE 1.4.   Basic structure of an immunoglobulin molecule. The antigen-binding sites (one of which is boxed off) are formed by the juxtaposition of variable regions of the heavy and light chains (V_H and V_L) in the Fab region of the molecule. Within these regions are hypervariable regions containing the antigen-binding cleft. Regions of the heavy and light chains with a relatively constant structure are indicated as C_{H1-3} and C_L. The Fc portion of the molecule contains the binding sites for complement proteins and inflammatory cells that contain Fc receptors. (Reprinted with permission from AK Abbas, AH Lichtman, JS Pober. Cellular and Molecular Immunology [3rd ed]. Philadelphia: Saunders, 1997;42.)

ADCC occurs when an antibody molecule bound to a target-cell antigen subsequently binds its Fc portion to an immune cell with an Fc receptor. Cells capable of such binding include macrophages, neutrophils, eosinophils, and NK cells. After binding, the immune cells secrete cytolytic factors that lyse the target. This mechanism has been shown to play a role in the elimination of IgE-bound parasites by eosinophils and in autoimmune thyroiditis. The role of antibodies in hypersensitivity reactions is discussed below. Neonatal immunity is mediated by maternal IgG that crosses the placenta.

No discussion of antibodies would be complete without at least touching on the experimental and clinical importance of monoclonal antibodies. These antibodies are produced by immortalized antibody-secreting cells that are created by the Nobel Prize–winning approach of Kohler and Milstein. Monoclonal antibodies have been used experimentally to identify and help characterize phenotypic markers on cells and for the purposes of diagnosis of infectious and tumor disease. In the clinical arena, they have been used therapeutically in a variety of scenarios including the elimination of cancerous tumors, the blockage of the effects of harmful cytokines, and for specific immunosuppression in transplantation.

Cytokines

The effector phase of adaptive immunity and the equivalent stage of innate immunity are carried out in large part by low-molecular-weight protein hormones called *cytokines*. These proteins are initially produced during the activation phase of lymphocyte stimulation and are also produced by APCs. Cytokines have pleiotropic effects, acting on many different cell types, and can have multiple effects on these cells. Cytokines can influence the secretion of other cytokines, and the actions of many cytokines are redundant.

A discussion of cytokines can rapidly become confusing because of the diversity of different types and because they tend to have overlapping functions. The approach taken here emulates that of Abbas et al. In their text on cellular immunology, they organized their discussion of the topic by grouping the cytokines into three different categories: cytokines that mediate and regulate innate immunity, cytokines that mediate and regulate specific immunity, and cytokines that stimulate hematopoiesis. To be succinct, only the most prominent cytokines in each group are discussed.

Cytokines That Mediate
and Regulate Innate Immunity

Type I Interferon.   Type I IFN consists of IFN-α and IFN-β and plays a role in inhibiting viral replication by inducing the formation of antiviral enzymes in infected cells. It also facilitates the lysis of virally infected cells by cytotoxic T lymphocytes by increasing target cell expression of class I MHC molecules and increases the lytic potential of NK cells.

Tumor Necrosis Factor.   Gram-negative bacteria, such as *Neisseria*, have lipopolysaccharide (LPS) in their cell walls. The principal cytokine released by macrophages in reaction to LPS during an infection with gram-negative bacteria is tumor necrosis factor (TNF). When released in appropriate amounts in response to infection, TNF induces endothelial cells at the infection site to express adhesion molecules, a subset of which are referred to as *integrins*. These molecules bind to ligands on lymphocytes, monocytes, and neutrophils and facilitate their recruitment into the area. TNF also activates these cells, making them better able to eliminate the triggering pathogen.

In fulminating infections, high levels of TNF can be produced that enter the blood and mediate systemic effects including fever, as well as wasting of muscle and fat tissue called *cachexia* that occurs as a result of TNF-induced appetite suppression. Cachexia is also seen in parasitic diseases and in AIDS, though in AIDS the pathogenesis is unclear. In gram-negative sepsis, when bacteria are disseminated widely through the circulation, massive quantities of TNF are produced which can lead to blood vessel coagulation and a reduction in blood pressure leading to septic shock and death. A number of clinical trials have attempted to treat septic shock by inhibiting TNF by using monoclonal antibodies directed against TNF itself or its receptor. Although the data are conflicting and disappointing, the validity of the approach is sound and success may depend on dosage and timing.

Interleukin-1.   The effects of interleukin-1 (IL-1) in innate immunity are similar to those described for TNF, and IL-1 can be produced by many more cell types. Virtually all body cells have receptors for IL-1 and can respond to it. There are two forms of IL-1, IL-1α and IL-1β, the latter of which uses IL-1 converting enzyme (ICE) for its production.[2] IL-1 is unique among cytokines in that there exist naturally occurring IL-1 inhibitors, the best characterized of which is IL-1 receptor antagonist (IL-1ra). Interestingly, IL-1ra was shown to be produced by unstimulated conjunctival epithelial cells.

Chemokines.   Chemokines are a family of chemotactic cytokines. There are two main subfamilies classified by their amino terminal structure. Both groups have two cysteine residues at their amino terminal end, but in one group, these residues are separated by another amino acid. The group in which the terminal cysteines are adjacent is referred to as *C-C chemokines*, and those in which another amino acid separates them is called the *C-X-C group*. C-C chemokines are preferentially secreted by T cells and act on T cells, monocytes, eosinophils, and basophils. Examples of this type include RANTES (regulated by activation, normal T cell expressed and secreted), macrophage inflammatory protein–1α and –1β (MIP-1α and MIP-1β), and eotaxin, all of which differ in their ability to recruit different cell types. C-X-C chemokines are produced by mononuclear phagocytes, endothelial cells, fibroblasts, and megakaryocytes and act predominantly on neutrophils. IL-8 and its functionally homologous chemokine MIP-2 are involved in neutrophil chemotaxis and are examples of C-X-C chemokines. Certain chemokine receptors were shown to act as coreceptors for the human immunodeficiency virus (HIV).

Defensins.   Defensins are small cationic peptides found in phagocytes and the intestinal mucosa that exert a wide range of antimicrobial activities through membrane permeabilization.[3] They electrostatically bind to membranes and then form multimeric pores. In addition to lysing microbes, they are thought to play a role in tissue inflammation and endocrine regulation during infection.[4]

*Cytokines That Mediate
and Regulate Specific Immunity*

Interleukin-1 and Interleukin-2.   Although IL-1 mediates aspects of innate immunity, it also plays an important immunoregulatory role in specific immunity by promoting the production of, and response to, IL-2 by T cells during T cell activation and by enhancing the growth of B cells. When an APC presents antigen to CD4+ T cells, it simultaneously secretes IL-1, which facilitates the expression of IL-2 receptors on the T cells; the T cells themselves also secrete IL-1. Following activation, T cells secrete IL-2, which binds to their own IL-2 receptors as well as those on neighboring activated cells (Figure 1.5). IL-2 is the principal cytokine responsible for the propagation of the immune response. It induces T cells to proliferate and promotes the production of other cytokines, such as IFN-γ, by T cells. It also promotes the growth of, and release of antibody by, B cells, and enhances the cytolytic potential of NK cells. This latter effect is the basis behind some antitumor therapies that rely on the injection of patient lymphocytes that have been precultured with high concentrations of IL-2 to stimulate their killing potential; these cells have been referred to as *lymphokine-activated killer* (LAK) *cells.*

Interleukin-4.   IL-4 is secreted by, and acts as a growth and differentiation factor for, Th2 cells, and is the chief cytokine involved in the secretion of antibody by B cells in response to T-dependent antigens. It plays an important role specifically in the production of IgE by B cells by inducing the isotype switch to IgE and thus is an important regulator of mast cell and eosinophil function. Mast cells use cell-bound IgE as a trigger for granule release in the allergic response, and both cell types mediate antiparasitic immunity by involving IgE in ADCC-type reactions.

Interferon-gamma.   IFN-γ, also called *type II IFN*, is produced by CD4+ and CD8+ T cells and NK cells, and plays a very important role in various aspects of cell-mediated immunity. First and foremost, IFN-γ is a potent

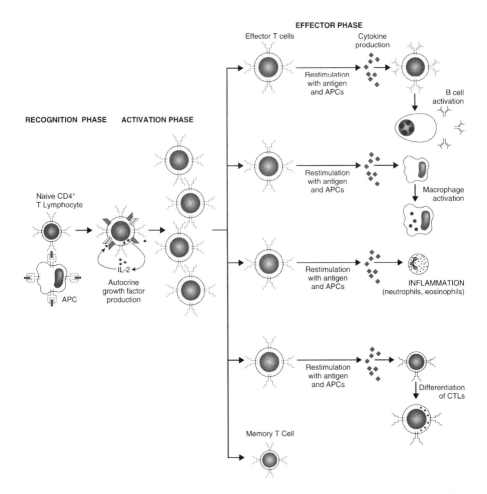

FIGURE 1.5.   Functional responses of T cells. Antigen recognition by a T cell (in this example, a CD4+ T cell) leads to IL-2 production, proliferation as a result of autocrine IL-2 stimulation, and effector cell functions (e.g., B cell stimulation, macrophage activation, promotion of inflammation, and help for cytotoxic T cell [CTL] differentiation). (APC = antigen-presenting cell.) (Reprinted with permission from AK Abbas, AH Lichtman, JS Pober. Cellular and Molecular Immunology [3rd ed]. Philadelphia: Saunders, 1997;140.)

activator of mononuclear phagocytes and belongs in the category of factors referred to as *macrophage-activating factors* (MAFs). Other effects include upregulation of class I and II MHC antigens on the surface of cells thus facilitating immune system recognition of foreign epitopes. The importance of the release of IFN-γ in response to intracellular infection (a Th1 response) is corroborated by the massively increased bacterial load and lethal disease that is seen in IFN-γ knockout mice in which the gene for this cytokine is deleted. In the eye, IFN-γ was shown to similarly enhance MHC antigen expression and induce recruitment of antigen-presenting Langerhans' cells into the central cornea, a region normally devoid of these cells. The implications of this in corneal disease are discussed in a later chapter.

Transforming Growth Factor–Beta.   Like many cytokines, transforming growth factor–beta (TGF-β) was named for its first demonstrated effect, that is, the ability to facilitate the growth of normal cells in soft agar. Since then, a host of other functions have been attributed to this factor, many of them immune functions. TGF-β inhibits the proliferation of T and B cells and the maturation of cytotoxic T cells but does not block the activity of cytotoxic T cells. It inhibits the activity of NK cells and macrophages. The effects of proinflammatory cytokines such as TNF on endothelial cells and neutrophils are also inhibited by TGF-β and have led to the characterization of TGF-β as an anticytokine. However, all of TGF-β's immune effects are not inhibitory, as just alluded to with regard to cytotoxic T cell activity. It attracts and activates monocytes and plays a role in inducing the switch to the IgA isotype in B cells. TGF-β plays an important role in intraocular immunity (discussed in Chapter 2), where it seems to be primarily responsible for mediating the phenomenon referred to as *anterior chamber–associated immune deviation* (ACAID).

Cytokines That Stimulate Hematopoiesis

A host of cytokines have been implicated in leukocyte growth and differentiation, including IL-3 and IL-7 and the colony-stimulating factors GM-CSF (granulocyte-monocyte CSF), M-CSF (monocyte CSF), and G-CSF (granulocyte CSF). These cytokines are released by both stromal and T cells in the marrow.

Regulation of the Immune Response

Several mechanisms play a role in downregulating the immune response after antigen activation. One contributing mechanism is simply the absence of antigen-induced immune stimulation following the elimination of antigen. Because many products of lymphocyte activation, such as antibodies and cytokines, are short-lived and are secreted for only brief periods after cell stimulation, the absence of antigenic stimulation ultimately results in the elimination of these effector molecules. Effector cells, such as plasma cells, are relatively short-lived and not self-renewing.

In addition to antigen elimination, the immune system has evolved a number of regulatory mechanisms to downregulate the immune response.

These include the development of suppressor T cells, antibody feedback, and Fas/Fas ligand (FasL) interactions.

Suppressor T Cells

Suppressor T cells do not appear to be a unique subset of cells but rather may represent different subsets of helper T cells that use a host of different mechanisms to inhibit immune responsiveness. These mechanisms include the localized release of TGF-β and the shift in T helper cell subset. In the latter case, a shift to a Th2 helper cell from a Th1 downregulates cell-mediated immunity and delayed-type hypersensitivity whereas a shift from a Th2 to a Th1 type may suppress IgE production in allergy by interfering with IL-4-mediated isotype switching to IgE.

Antibody Feedback

Antibodies play an important role in adaptive immunity by preventing intracellular infection by eliminating and neutralizing antigens. Antibodies also play a role in limiting the activity of B cells by a mechanism referred to as antibody feedback. In this process, antigen-bound antibody attaches to the surface of the activated B cell by binding to its Fc receptor and becomes situated adjacent to the B cell's immunoglobulin antigen receptor. When this occurs, antigen receptor cross-linking results, inducing an intracellular stop signal which inhibits the production of more antibody.

Fas/Fas Ligand Interactions

Fas was originally described as a cell surface molecule that could mediate apoptotic cell death. Activated lymphocytes have Fas as well as the binding ligand of Fas, called *FasL*, on their cell surface. Among their other functions, it has been speculated that these molecules play a role in regulating immune reactions following the elimination of antigen. As the level of antigen wanes, the probability increases that Fas on one lymphocyte will bind to FasL on another; when this occurs, the Fas-containing cell undergoes apoptotic cell death. This is an effective mechanism that results in the reduction in effector cell numbers (Figure 1.6).

Hypersensitivity Reactions

The term *hypersensitivity* applies to adaptive immune reactions that are exaggerated or inappropriately active, resulting in tissue damage. These reactions generally occur after secondary exposure to antigen. There are five types of hypersensitivity reactions, most of which have been observed in the eye. The original classification of hypersensitivity reactions by Coombs and Gell described four types, but a fifth has been added. A summary of the classification of hypersensitivity reactions appears in Table 1.3.

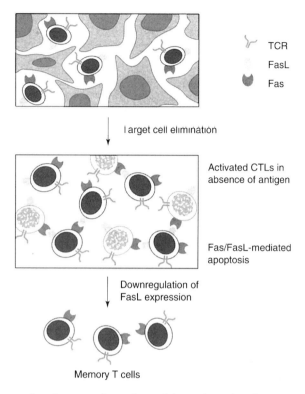

FIGURE 1.6. Role of Fas and Fas ligand (FasL) in the downregulation of the immune response to antigen. As the number of antigenic target cells wanes, the probability of T-T cell interaction increases, promoting the binding of Fas on one cell to the FasL on another. Such binding results in the apoptotic death of the Fas-containing cell. (TCR = T cell surface antigen receptor; CTLs = cytotoxic T cells.) (Reprinted with permission from DH Lynch, R Ramsdell, MR Alderson. Fas and FasL in the homeostatic regulation of immune responses. Immunol Today 1995;16:569–574. Copyright 1995, with permission from Elsevier Science.)

Type I: Immediate Hypersensitivity

Type I hypersensitivity is triggered within minutes in response to environmental antigens such as pollens, mold spores, feces of dust mites, and animal dander. The classic example of a type I reaction in the eye is seasonal allergic conjunctivitis. After it has entered the body, an allergen binds to a B cell, which processes it, incorporates it in the context of its surface class II MHC molecules, and then presents it to Th2 cells (note that in this activation scenario, B cells act as APCs). Successful activation of Th2 cells by B cell antigen presentation requires the expression of costimulators such as B7 and CD40, which bind to CD28 and CD40 ligand on the T cell, respectively. The stimulated Th2 cell then releases IL-4 and IL-13, which induce

TABLE 1.3
Classification of Hypersensitivity Reactions

Type of Hypersensitivity	Mediators	Effector Mechanism
I: Immediate	IgE	Mast cell mediator release
II: Antibody-mediated	IgM and IgG	Complement proteins Inflammatory cell mediators Opsonization Antibody-dependent cell- mediated cytotoxicity
III: Immune complex disease	IgM and IgG immune complexes	Complement proteins Inflammatory cell mediators
IV: Delayed-type	APCs, CD4+ and CD8+ T cells	Activated macrophages
V: Activating antibodies	Antihormone receptor antibody	Activation of target cell

an isotype switch to IgE in the B cell. Similar activation of the Th2 cell likely occurs by direct presentation by APCs that have also processed the antigen. IgE is released by the B cell and binds by its Fc region to a receptor on the surface of mast cells. On re-exposure, the antigen binds to the Fab region of mast cell–bound IgE, cross-linking adjacent molecules. This quickly leads to the activation of protein kinase C, which phosphorylates myosin light chains and leads to the disassembly of actin-myosin complexes beneath the plasma membrane, resulting in the release of mast cell granules containing histamine and heparin.

Mast cell activation also results in the activation of phospholipase A_2, both directly and indirectly, through an induced elevation in intracellular Ca^{++} that catalyzes the liberation of membrane arachidonic acid. Arachidonic acid is then converted to leukotrienes (LTB_4, LTC_4, LTD_4, and LTE_4), prostaglandins (PGD_2), and platelet-activating factors (PAF), under the influence of lipoxygenase, cyclooxygenase, and acetyl transferase enzymes, respectively (Figure 1.7). Collectively, the preformed and newly formed mediators act as chemoattractants and vasodilators, and they increase vascular permeability.

After several hours, a late phase of this reaction occurs that is mediated by the release of TNF and IL-1 by mast cells as well as IL-5 from Th2 cells. Under the influence of these cytokines, T cells (primarily of the Th2 type), eosinophils, and basophils accumulate at the site of antigen exposure. An example of a late-phase reaction is eczema, or atopic dermatitis.

Asthma represents a late-phase reaction in the lungs that results in smooth muscle hypertrophy and hyperactivity triggered by the release of

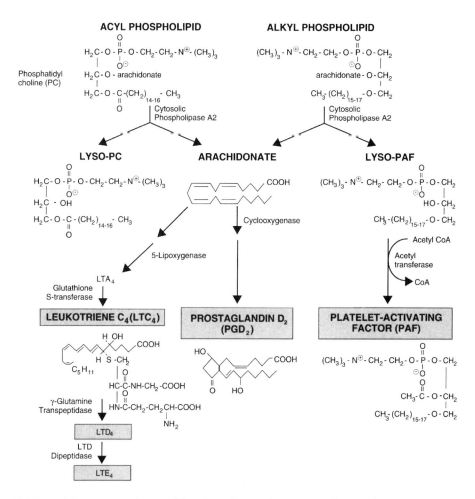

FIGURE 1.7.   Biosynthesis of lipid mediators by mast cells. Breakdown of membrane phospholipids by cytosolic phospholipase A2 leads to generation of leukotriene C_4, prostaglandin D_2, and platelet-activating factor. (Reprinted with permission from AK Abbas, AH Lichtman, JS Pober. Cellular and Molecular Immunology [3rd ed]. Philadelphia: Saunders, 1997;308.)

factors from accumulating leukocytes. The leukotriene LTC_4 and its breakdown products (LTD_4 and LTE_4) and PAF are released from mast cells in the lungs and play an important role in mediating bronchoconstriction. Mucosal mast cells in the lungs do not release appreciable amounts of histamine, and as a result, antihistamines are ineffective in the treatment of this condition. The ability of the mast cell mediator tryptase to degrade the bronchodilator vasoactive intestinal polypeptide in the lung could be yet another mechanism for allergy-induced bronchoconstriction.[5]

Type II: Antibody-Mediated Hypersensitivity

Antibody-binding reactions play a role in mediating type II hypersensitivity. There are four basic effector mechanisms in which antibody is involved.

1. Classical pathway complement activation resulting in the osmotic lysis of the target.
2. Recruitment and activation of inflammatory cells. This process also begins with the activation of complement proteins but results not in target lysis but in the local generation of complement chemotactic proteins such as C5a, which recruit inflammatory cells into an area of inflammation. The release by these cells of hydrolytic enzymes, reactive oxygen-free radicals, leukotrienes, prostaglandins, and other cytokines, contributes to inflammation.
3. Phagocytosis of antibody-coated cells. In this scenario, antibodies act as opsonins, facilitating the uptake and destruction of target antigens by phagocytic cells by the process of opsonization.
4. The ADCC reaction is mediated by NK cells that bind to cell-bound antibodies and release cytotoxic mediators that destroy the target cell.

Complement-Mediated Cell Lysis

Examples of hypersensitivity reactions that involve complement-mediated cell lysis include the transfusion reaction, hemolytic disease of the newborn, and hyperacute graft rejection. A transfusion reaction occurs when donor/recipient blood types are mismatched. Serum from individuals with blood type O, which lacks A and B blood group antigens, agglutinates red blood cells bearing these antigens. Similarly, serum from individuals with blood type A agglutinates red cells from donors with blood type B, and serum from individuals with blood type B agglutinates red cells from donors with blood type A. Agglutination is mediated by antibodies present in the serum.

Individuals with blood type O have antibodies to both antigens A and B, whereas type A individuals have antibodies to B and type B individuals have antibodies to A. These antibodies develop before exposure to foreign blood types because the immune system is exposed to them in other venues, such as on intestinal flora. Subjects with blood type A are tolerant of this antigen and therefore do not develop antibodies to antigen A that their immune system later encounters in the gut, but rather only to B; the converse is true for people with blood type B. Individuals with type O have not been rendered tolerant to either types A or B and thus develop antibodies to both. Because the red cells in type O blood lack surface antigens A and B, these cells can be transfused without adverse consequences into people with type A or B blood. On the other hand, individuals with type AB blood will express both antigens on their cells, will have been made tolerant to them, and will not express antibodies to A and B antigens. These individuals will be able to accept blood from individuals with types A, B, and O. All other matchups other than between identical types would result in antibody-mediated agglutination of donor red blood cells, accompanied by complement activation and intravascular hemolysis (destruction of red blood cells). Red blood cell destruction may cause circulatory shock, and the released contents of the red cells can produce acute tubular necrosis in the kidney.

In hemolytic disease of the newborn, a mother develops IgG antibodies to blood group antigens on the fetus. IgG crosses the placenta and lyses the fetal cells harboring the antigens by a complement-dependent lytic mechanism. Rhesus D (RhD) is the most common antigen involved in this disease. A risk arises when an Rh– mother carries an Rh+ infant. Sensitization of the Rh– mother to the Rh+ red cells usually occurs during birth when some fetal red cells enter the maternal circulation. While a first child is unaffected by this condition, all successive children have an increasing risk of being affected.

To avoid Rh-mediated disease, the mother is injected with anti-Rh antibodies (Rhogam) immediately following her first delivery. These antibodies destroy and remove any residual Rh antigens in the maternal circulation, thus preventing them from stimulating a maternal immune response. They may also serve to inhibit maternal B cells that have been activated by the antigen by the mechanism of antibody feedback described above.

In hyperacute rejection, rapid thrombotic occlusion of the graft vasculature begins within minutes after host vessels are engrafted. This form of rejection is mediated by pre-existing complement-fixing antibodies that bind to, and damage, endothelial cells, causing them to secrete factors that result in platelet aggregation and coagulation. This process results in vascular occlusion and irreversible organ damage.

Recruitment and Activation of Inflammatory Cells

Two things occur after inflammatory phagocytic cells are recruited into an area of inflammation: either they phagocytose the offending antigen or, if the antigen is too large, they release their harmful mediators extracellularly. It is this latter case that forms the basis of this subset of type II hypersensitivity. Examples of this type of reaction include Goodpasture's syndrome, cicatricial pemphigoid, and Mooren's ulcer. In Goodpasture's syndrome, patients express autoantibodies to a glycoprotein in the glomerular basement membrane. This antibody is of the IgG type which activates complement, resulting in the recruitment of inflammatory cells. These cells are unable to phagocytose the inducing basement membrane antigens and therefore release their toxic mediators extracellularly in an attempt to destroy and eliminate them. The battlefield equivalent of this scenario is "carpet bombing." The extracellular release of these mediators usually results in severe necrosis of the glomerulus. Lung damage also occurs in these patients because the basement membrane in the alveoli contains autoantigens to which the above antibody cross-reacts.

In cicatricial pemphigoid and Mooren's ulcer, autoantibodies involved in the recruitment of destructive inflammatory cells develop to different conjunctival and corneal epithelial antigens. These are discussed in more detail in Chapter 5.

Phagocytosis of Antibody-Coated Cells

In autoimmune hemolytic anemia, patients produce antibodies to their own red blood cells. These opsonized cells are phagocytosed by macrophages in the liver and spleen, leading to the depletion of erythrocytes and anemia.

Antibody-Dependent Cell-Mediated Cytotoxicity

ADCC has been postulated to play a role in the tissue damage that occurs in autoimmune thyroiditis, that is, inflammation of the thyroid gland.

Type III: Immune Complex Disease

Under the right conditions of stimulation with a divalent or multivalent antigen (an antigen with at least two identical antigenic sequences), antigen-antibody, or immune, complexes form. These complexes are generally removed effectively by the mononuclear phagocyte system. However, under certain conditions, their presence persists and can trigger a hypersensitivity reaction. Three important sets of circumstances, as outlined by Roitt et al.,[6] are most conducive to the formation of dangerous amounts of immune complexes.

1. Persistent low-grade infection by various microorganisms—for example, certain streptococcal and staphylococcal bacteria, parasites, or viruses such as those that cause hepatitis—leads to chronic immune complex formation, facilitating their eventual deposition in the tissues.
2. In autoimmunity, continued production of autoantibody to (persistent) self-antigens leads to prolonged immune complex formation and deposition.
3. Immune complexes may be formed at body surfaces. For example, lung deposition may occur following repeated inhalation of antigenic materials such as moldy hay in farmers (i.e., farmer's lung disease) or animal dander in animal care technicians.

Factors Influencing Immune Complex Deposition

Several factors determine the extent of immune complex deposition:

1. Intermediate-sized complexes appear to be most prone to deposition.
2. Accumulation of complexes is inversely proportional to the ability of the host to clear them from the circulation. Removal is carried out by mononuclear phagocytes in the liver and spleen. Complement also plays a role by solubilizing and breaking down large complexes.

TABLE 1.4
Factors Influencing the Precipitation of Immune Complexes

Size: intermediate-sized complexes most readily precipitate
Rate of clearance: precipitation is inversely related to clearance
Antigenic charge: cationic antigens are drawn to anionic sites (e.g., glomerular
  basement membrane)
Vessel structure: tortuosity facilitates complex trapping
Vessel hemodynamics: high pressure promotes complex trapping

Specifically, complement-mediated removal is accomplished by the binding of complement to the complexes and its subsequent binding to red cells by way of erythrocyte complement receptors; these cells are then removed by hepatic macrophages.

3. Complexes containing cationic antibodies or antigens bind avidly to negatively charged components, for example, in the glomerular basement membrane. Cationic immunoglobulins bind to anionic sites in the uveal connective tissue and can complex, in situ, with antigen.

4. Anatomic and hemodynamic factors are important. Capillaries such as those in the renal glomeruli, synovia, and ciliary bodies, which are sites of immune complex deposition, ultrafilter the plasma under pressure to produce urine, synovial fluid, and aqueous humor, respectively. Even nonfiltering capillaries are susceptible to this disease if they follow a tortuous course; immune complexes tend to be pushed into the walls of such vessels by centrifugal force.

A summary of the factors influencing immune complex deposition appears in Table 1.4.

Mechanism of Immune Complex Disease

Immune complexes are usually phagocytosed and cleared by macrophages in the liver and spleen. In high concentrations, immune complexes deposit in the tissues where they activate complement leading to the recruitment and activation of inflammatory cells, predominantly neutrophils, at the sites of immune complex deposition. These cells then cause tissue injury by the "carpet bombing" mechanism described above (Figure 1.8). Because the complexes deposit mainly in arterioles, particularly in the renal glomeruli and joint synovia, the clinical and pathologic manifestations are vasculitis, nephritis, and arthritis.

Examples of Immune Complex Diseases

As mentioned above, the glomerulus, synovial membrane, ciliary body, and other regions where there is vascular tortuosity are susceptible to

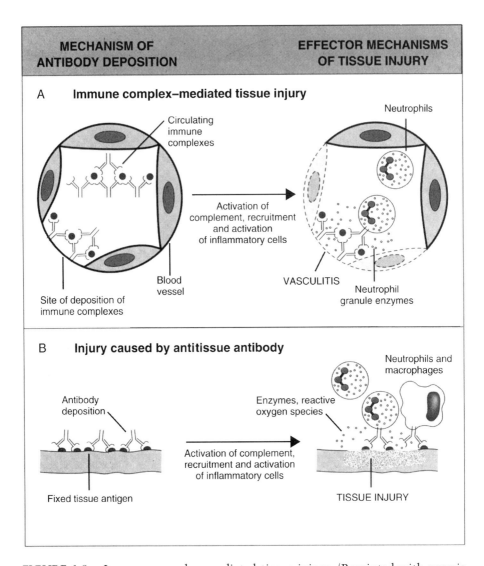

FIGURE 1.8.   Immune complex–mediated tissue injury. (Reprinted with permission from AK Abbas, AH Lichtman, JS Pober. Cellular and Molecular Immunology [3rd ed]. Philadelphia: Saunders, 1997;426.)

immune complex–mediated inflammation. Systemic examples of diseases that are thought to have sequelae resulting from complex deposition include systemic lupus erythematosus; poststreptococcal glomerulonephritis, which develops after throat infections with this microbe; and polyarteritis nodosa, which occurs as a consequence of hepatitis B infection. Ocular immune complex disease manifests itself as peripheral corneal lesions in rheumatoid arthritis, uveitis in Crohn's disease, and retinochoroiditis in *Toxoplasma* infection, among others.

Type IV: Delayed-Type Hypersensitivity

Delayed-type hypersensitivity (DTH) reactions are hypersensitivity reactions to protein antigens and take more than 12 hours to develop. Unlike other forms of hypersensitivity, DTH cannot be transferred by serum but can be transferred by T lymphocytes that have become sensitized to a particular antigen. These cells act in concert with other cell types that are recruited to the site of the reaction.

There are two types of DTH reactions: contact hypersensitivity (CH; also called *contact dermatitis*) and the tuberculin reaction. CH is restricted to the epidermal layer and is characterized by the development of eczema (dermatitis) approximately 48 hours after exposure to antigen. Allergens that induce this type of reaction include poison ivy, poison oak, rubber, and metals such as nickel and chromate. Some of these are not in and of themselves antigenic but become so after being conjugated to normal body proteins. Initial immune cell infiltration into the area occurs around 3 hours after exposure and consists of T cells and macrophages seen around the local vasculature in the dermis. This is followed by infiltration of these cells into the epidermis where they act to eliminate the antigen over the next 2–3 days.

The tuberculin reaction is induced by soluble antigens from a number of organisms, including *Mycobacterium* and *Listeria*. The localized cutaneous reaction to these antigens is used as the basis for a test of exposure to these organisms, for example the TB test in the case of tuberculosis. As in contact hypersensitivity, T cells and macrophages play a role in antigen elimination, but in the tuberculin reaction, these cells remain in the dermis. Induration (hardness) is the hallmark of the tuberculin reaction, which is generally maximal at 48 hours.

Sequence of Events in a Delayed-Type
Hypersensitivity Reaction

Specialized resident APCs in the epidermis (i.e., Langerhans' cells) process antigen and migrate to draining lymph nodes where they present antigenic epitopes to T cells, activating them. Langerhans' cells are thought to present antigen for initial immunization only. The activated T cells then migrate back to the site of antigen entry and secrete inflammatory cytokines such as TNF, which activate neighboring endothelial cells. These endothelial cells respond by producing vasodilator substances such as prostacyclin and nitric oxide, resulting in increased blood flow to the area. The endothelium also changes shape, facilitating leakage of plasma and cells into the underlying tissue; they also secrete or express chemotactic factors such as IL-8 and the adhesion molecules E-selectin, vascular cell adhesion molecule–1

(VCAM-1), and ICAM-1. These adhesion molecules promote neutrophil, lymphocyte, and monocyte recruitment, respectively.

Macrophages are the final effector cells in the DTH reaction. In response to IFN-γ released by activated Th1 and CD8+ T cells, these macrophages become activated to become more efficient phagocytes and play a critical role in the resolution of DTH. Some microbes are resistant to the cytocidal effects of activated macrophages. In such cases, a chronic DTH reaction can occur resulting in the fusion of the chronically activated macrophages around the offending organism; these cells are then referred to as *multinucleated giant cells*. Macrophages may also interconnect with each other in a manner resembling an epithelium in an attempt to wall off the area of infection; in this case, the macrophages are referred to as *epithelioid cells*. Both types of these macrophages secrete factors that result in tissue fibrosis, resulting in the formation of a granuloma that typically has a nodular appearance. This excessive fibrosis damages neighboring tissue and compromises function. The spot on a tuberculous lung is a granuloma. It is only when the offending antigen is eliminated that the process abates. (In the case of tuberculosis, the administration of a new generation of potent antibiotics was necessary to accomplish this.)

Examples of Type IV Hypersensitivity Diseases

DTH plays a role in ocular allergy, as well as in corneal graft rejection, cosmetic-induced conjunctivitis, idiopathic uveitis, and sympathetic ophthalmia. A host of systemic autoimmune diseases, such as type I diabetes, encephalomyelitis, and Crohn's disease, also have an important DTH component.

Type V

An addition to the four classic types of hypersensitivity is *type V hypersensitivity*. This reaction is mediated by antibodies that bind to surface hormone receptors and activate, rather than block, intracellular signaling. The best example of this is the effect of thyroid-stimulating autoantibody on the thyroid-stimulating hormone receptor on thyrocytes in Graves' disease. Binding of these antibodies activates adenyl cyclase, which ultimately results in the release of high levels of thyroid hormone.

Transplantation

Transplantation refers to the process by which cells, tissues, or organs are taken from one individual and placed into another. The transplanted item, referred to as a *graft*, is obtained from a donor and is transplanted into a recipient or host. The transplantation of an organ (or cells or tissue) into a non–MHC-matched, nonimmunosuppressed recipient will be immunologically rejected by the host. Such grafts are referred to as *allogeneic grafts* or *allografts*. Tissue grafts taken from a donor who is a genetic twin of the host is referred to as a *syngeneic graft* or *syngraft* and is not rejected. Tissues removed and then engrafted back into the same individual are referred to as *autografts* or *autologous grafts*. Examples include skin for burn victims, venous grafts in coronary bypass patients, and bone marrow grafts in certain cancer patients. *Xenografts* are obtained from a different donor species and are rejected.

Mechanisms of Solid Graft Rejection

Three mechanisms play a role in graft rejection. The first mechanism is referred to as *hyperacute graft rejection* and is an example of a type II hypersensitivity reaction. In this type of rejection, alloantibodies bind to ABO blood group antigens on endothelial cells and activate complement, resulting in the release of thrombotic factors that cause vascular occlusion and graft necrosis within minutes. Because all donors and recipients are typed before transplantation, this reaction no longer occurs in human allografts. It is an issue in xenoengraftment, however, in which the host possesses natural antibodies to various donor determinants. Other target antigens on allografted endothelial cells that play a role in hyperacute rejection are foreign MHC molecules to which the recipient may have been exposed through blood transfusion or multiple pregnancies.

Acute vascular rejection has a similar outcome as hyperacute rejection, but it occurs by a slightly different mechanism. In this case, antibodies against endothelial alloantigens, such as MHC antigens, activate complement, resulting in recruitment of inflammatory cells including T cells, which induce a severe vasculitis and necrosis. This type of rejection occurs about a week after transplantation. Acute cellular rejection begins after the first week and is mediated by a DTH mechanism, as well as by the activity of cytotoxic T cells directed against foreign MHC antigens on the parenchymal cells in the transplanted organ.

Molecular Basis of Allorecognition in Acute Cellular Rejection

Two theories have been postulated to explain the mechanism of cell-mediated alloreactivity. According to the first, referred to as *direct presentation*, alloreactive host T cells respond, by way of their TCR, directly to foreign MHC molecules on passenger leukocytes or parenchymal cells in the allograft. It has been speculated that some of these alloreactive host T cells may in fact be responding to foreign MHC molecules, which have incorporated a peptide common to the host and donor but to which the host has not developed tolerance because it did not fit into the host's MHC antigen binding groove. In the second scenario, called *indirect presentation*, peptide antigens derived from the graft become associated, after processing, with host MHC molecules on APCs and are presented to host T cells.

In Vitro Measurement of Histocompatibility

One way to quantitate histocompatibility between a donor and recipient is to co-culture their peripheral blood cells in a mixed lymphocyte reaction. The donor cells are pretreated with antimitotic drugs to prevent them from proliferating and responding to the recipient's cells; this allows for the measurement of only the response of the recipient to the donor. If there are differences in the MHC alleles between the donor and recipient, a large proportion of the recipient's leukocytes will become activated and will proliferate over the ensuing 4 days. The magnitude of this response is measured by quantifying the accumulation of ^{3}H-thymidine into the DNA of the replicating cells.

Prevention of Allograft Rejection

The most important strategy for the prevention of allograft rejection is to minimize the MHC incompatibility of the donor and recipient. The only exception to this appears to be in corneal transplantation, in which the data suggest that non–MHC-matched grafts experience the same rejection rate as matched grafts, probably due to the immunologically privileged nature of the cornea.

Other approaches being explored in animal models include the removal of donor passenger lymphocytes from the graft and the induction of immunologic tolerance to the foreign antigen. The removal of passenger cells from pancreatic islets of Langerhans and thyroid grafts has shown promising results in animals. Attempts have been made to induce tolerance to allografts by interfering with costimulatory signals, by T cell vaccination, and by administering donor immune cells intravenously to the recipient, bypassing draining lymph nodes. The success of this latter approach has been observed in human recipients of kidney allografts who were transfused with donor blood.

Despite attempts to match the donor and recipient as closely as possible, organ rejection still occurs. The use of highly effective immunosuppressive agents with limited side effects has prevented rejection in these patients and has transformed the field of transplantation. These agents include cyclosporin A, rapamycin, FK506, and OKT3. Cyclosporin A selectively blocks the transcription of IL-2 in activated T cells. FK506 is structurally unrelated to cyclosporin A but has a similar effect on T cells. Rapamycin blocks the signals induced by IL-2 binding to its receptor and thus inhibits T cell proliferation; it also has an inhibitory effect on B cells. OKT3 is a monoclonal antibody that binds to CD3, which is an accessory molecule located near the TCR and acts in conjunction with it to cause T cell activation. Binding of OKT3 ultimately results in the complement-mediated lysis of the T cell.

Graft-versus-Host Disease

Graft-versus-host (GVH) disease is a condition in which allogeneic donor lymphocytes react against tissues in an immunologically compromised host. A clinical situation in which this may occur is allogeneic bone marrow transplantation. This procedure is performed after an individual's own bone marrow is destroyed by radiation in an attempt to eliminate tumorous hematopoietic cells. It involves the injection into the recipient of closely matched donor bone marrow cells, which, it is hoped, will repopulate the marrow and start producing normal blood cells.

If there is sufficient histoincompatibility, donor immune cells will respond to immunogenic recipient antigens present on different target organs including the skin, liver, gastrointestinal tract, and lungs. These attacking donor cells would not be a threat if the recipient were not immunocompromised, because the recipient's immune cells would then be able to destroy the offending grafted cells. GVH disease appears to be mediated by alloreactive, immunocompetent donor T cells present in the donor marrow. Elimination of these cells has reduced bone marrow rejection but has also reduced the success of engraftment. This latter finding was thought to be due to the fact that T cells secrete hematopoietic factors that facilitate bone marrow cell growth.

Immunity to Tumors

Cancer is a general term used to describe a variety of different malignant neoplasms (new growths), most of which invade surrounding tissues and which often metastasize and grow at secondary sites. Cancers are given different names depending on their tissue type of origin. A malignant tumor derived from an epithelial cell is called a *carcinoma* and is the most common type. Malignant tumors of mesenchymal tissues, arising from fibroblasts, muscle, or fat cells are termed *sarcomas*. *Lymphomas* are solid malignant tumors of lymphoid tissues. *Leukemias* are marrow and blood-borne malignant tumors of lymphocytes and other hematopoietic cells. *Adenomas* are ordinarily benign epithelial tumors.

Tumor Antigens

A major surveillance function of the immune system is to recognize and destroy cancerous and precancerous cells before they grow into tumors. If malignant cells and tumors can stimulate an immune response, it follows that they express tumor antigens that are recognized by cells of the immune system. Tumor antigens may be uniquely expressed on a tumor cell or may be a normal cellular antigen that is simply overexpressed on the tumor. Antigens present only on tumor cells are referred to as *tumor-specific antigens*. Antigens expressed on both normal and tumor cells are referred to as *tumor-associated antigens*.

Some tumor antigens are specific for a particular tumor and represent normal differentiation antigens that happen to be overexpressed. Examples of these are certain antigens on melanoma cells and prostate-specific antigen on prostatic carcinoma cells. However, most tumor antigens studied are not unique but are shared by different tumors.

Certain tumor antigens, referred to as *oncofetal antigens*, are normally expressed on fetal but not adult tissues. Because these antigens were present during self-tolerance induction in early life, the immune system is unresponsive to them. The measurement of the level of these antigens in the blood of a cancer patient does have useful diagnostic and prognostic value, however. The two most thoroughly described oncofetal antigens are alpha-fetoprotein (AFP) and carcinoembryonic antigen (CEA). AFP may be significantly elevated in hepatocellular carcinoma, whereas CEA may be elevated in colon cancer.

Role of Viruses in Cancer

Some viruses have the ability to transform normal cells into cancer cells. Thus, the role of NK cells is important not only in ridding the body of newly formed tumors but also of potentially tumorigenic virally infected cells. Both RNA and DNA viruses have been implicated in the development of tumors. For example, DNA viruses implicated in the development of cancer are the Epstein-Barr virus (EBV) in certain lymphomas, human papillomavirus in cervical carcinoma, cytomegalovirus (CMV) in Kaposi's sarcoma, and hepatitis B virus in hepatocellular carcinoma. The only well-established human RNA tumor virus is human T lymphotropic virus–1 (HTLV-1), which has been implicated in T cell leukemia. Virally induced tumors usually express viral proteins, which are highly immunogenic, on their cell surface and serve as targets for the cell-mediated arm of the immune response.

Effector Mechanisms in Antitumor Immunity

In many cases, antibodies are produced to tumors, but there is little evidence for their direct role in inhibiting tumor development or growth. However, they may play a role in NK cell-mediated ADCC against tumors. Cytotoxic T cells play an important role in antitumor immunity. This is certainly not surprising for tumors expressing viral antigens because cytotoxic T cells normally play a role in lysing virally infected cells. The blood of patients with advanced tumors contains cytotoxic T cells capable of lysing tumor cells. Unlike classic cytotoxic T cells, NK cells do not recognize antigen in the context of MHC molecules, that is, they are not immunologically restricted. This is fortunate with regard to their role in directly killing tumor cells because tumor cells usually express very low levels of histocompatibility antigens. In fact, it may be the dearth of MHC surface antigens on tumor cells that make them uniquely recognizable to NK cells. As already mentioned, NK cells play a role in the surveillance and destruction of virally infected and transformed cells. Aside from directly lysing tumor cells, NK cells also lyse tumor cells by an ADCC mechanism.

Macrophages are also important cellular mediators of antitumor immunity. Like NK cells, macrophages can kill tumor cells by an ADCC mechanism. TNF plays an important role as the cytokine mediator of the direct and indirect tumor-killing effects of macrophages. TNF can kill tumor cells directly or indirectly by inducing thrombosis in tumor vessels.

Mechanisms of Evasion of the Immune System by Tumors

Knowledge of the way tumors evade the immune response is important to immunologists striving to develop unique approaches to therapy. Several of the existing mechanisms are as follows:

1. The tumor may express nonimmunogenic antigens, such as oncofetal antigens.
2. Cancer cells grow rapidly, allowing for the establishment of immunologically resistant tumors before an effective immune response can develop.
3. Some antitumor antibodies may facilitate tumor cell evasion of the immune response by denuding the surface of the cell of its antigens. This occurs as a result of the internalization of the surface antigen-antibody complex. The loss of surface expression of tumor antigens as a result of antibody binding is called *antigenic modulation*.
4. Tumor cells secrete factors that are themselves immunosuppressive. An example is TGF-β or factors similar to it, which is secreted in large amounts by many tumors. Recall that TGF-β is a potent inhibitor of T and B cell function.
5. Tumors that grow in the intraocular environment are not subject to the full immune system armamentarium because of suppressor factors in the aqueous humor and because of the phenomenon referred to as ACAID (see Chapter 2).

Immunotherapeutic Approaches for the Treatment of Cancer

The mainstay of cancer therapy for many years has been, and continues to be, the administration of chemotherapeutic agents that inhibit cell replication. The theory of this approach is that because tumor cells are fast-growing cells, they would preferentially succumb to treatments targeting the machinery of cell replication. Although the immune system and gastrointestinal tract, additional sites of rapid cell turnover, are also damaged, they would be expected to be replaced by available stem cells. In some cancers, however, this treatment only serves to select for tumor cells that are resistant to chemotherapy and that continue to grow.

Immunotherapy is the term used to define the treatment approaches that attempt to boost the immune system's response to cancer. The methodologies used have been diverse and have met with varying degrees of success. Examples include the following:

1. Injection of cancer patients with nonspecific immune stimulants called *adjuvants* at the sites of tumor growth. This approach was shown to boost macrophage-mediated destruction of tumor cells in a melanoma.
2. Treatment with type I IFN. This cytokine has been used with some success to treat various types of human cancers such as hairy cell leukemia, papillomas, Kaposi's sarcoma, renal carcinomas, and melanomas. IFN may exert its effects by activating NK cells and macrophages and possibly by directly inhibiting tumor cell growth. It may also make tumor cells more susceptible to cytotoxic T cell lysis by enhancing tumor cell histocompatibility antigen expression. It has been suggested that IFN, released during concomitant viral infections, may be responsible for the occasional remissions that are seen in these cancers.
3. Toxin-labeled monoclonal antibodies. In this approach, monoclonal antibodies directed against tumor antigens are attached to molecules that become toxic after they have been internalized by the tumor cell following antibody binding. Toxins that have been used include diphtheria and ricin (a plant toxin). Toxin-labeled anti–IL-2 receptor antibodies have been used for the treatment of T cell leukemias that express high levels of the receptor.
4. Injection of LAK cells. LAK cells are highly cytotoxic cells of NK and T cell origin produced by culture of these cells in high concentrations of IL-2. Injections of autologous LAK cells, coupled with infusions of IL-2, have been shown to cause remissions in patients with melanoma and kidney tumors. Some approaches have used tumor infiltrating lymphocytes for the production of LAK cells.
5. Photodynamic therapy. This treatment modality is being explored as an option in surface tumors such as skin cancers. It involves the administration of a compound that is preferentially taken up by tumor cells and that is rendered toxic by treatment with a laser.

Autoimmunity

Autoimmune diseases develop when the immune system attacks the body's own cells, tissues, or organs. Systemic autoimmune diseases, characterized by multiple autoimmune phenomena, are a result of the activation of numerous clones of lymphocytes directed against a host of different self-antigens. In contrast, organ-specific autoimmune diseases are characterized by the activation of lymphocytes that are reactive against only a limited number of self-antigens.

Mechanisms of Development of Autoimmunity

Several mechanisms may play a role in the development of autoimmunity, as follows:

1.   Autoimmunity may develop if self-reactive clones of lymphocytes fail to be deleted in the thymus.
2.   Autoreactive lymphocytes that survive but are normally unresponsive to self-antigens may be stimulated by cross-reactive foreign antigens. This cross-reactivity of foreign antigens with self-antigens, resulting in the initiation of an immune response against self-antigens, is referred to as *mimicry*.
3.   Self-antigens, not normally accessible and thus not rendered tolerant by the immune system, may become exposed for the first time, thereby initiating an immune response. This is particularly relevant to autoimmune eye diseases such as lens-induced uveitis and sympathetic ophthalmia.
4.   Regulatory mechanisms that normally prevent the activation of autoreactive lymphocytes that exist peripherally may be circumvented. Data suggest that a number of self-reactive clones are present in normal individuals but are actively suppressed. Polyclonal activators such as LPS in bacterial cell walls stimulate a large number of T or B cells irrespective of their antigenic specificity and thus have the potential to arouse a dormant self-reactive clone.

Genetic Factors in Autoimmunity

Although environmental factors such as exposure to cross-reacting microbes play an important role in autoimmunity, another strong predisposing factor is genetic makeup. Several genes have been implicated in autoimmunity, including those encoding the MHC, Fas, and as yet unknown genes that regulate cytokine expression.

HLA typing of large groups of patients with various autoimmune diseases has revealed a correlation between autoimmunity and certain histocompatibility alleles, many of which are class II alleles but some of which are class I. This fact has made it possible to estimate the relative risk of developing a disease based on an individual's HLA type.

Why should there be a correlation between histocompatibility type and autoimmunity? The answer is unknown, but at least three explanations have been postulated based on experimental data. One possibility is that certain MHC molecules show direct mimicry with microbial antigens. Another possibility is that certain histocompatibility types are inefficient in binding to, and rendering tolerant, developing thymic T cells. This results in the escape into the periphery of some autoreactive clones. Finally, it is also possible that MHC molecules may have different abilities to influence the development of regulatory cells.

Congenital and Acquired Immunodeficiencies

A host of different genetic defects, collectively referred to as *congenital immunodeficiencies*, negatively affect the body's ability to defend itself against infection and the growth of transformed cells. It is estimated that 500,000 people a year are born in the United States with a defect in some component of their immune system. Congenital immunodeficiencies can affect the activity of T and B cells, as well as macrophages and neutrophils. Immunodeficiencies that develop as a result of immune system infection (e.g., HIV), treatment with immunosuppressive drugs (e.g., to prevent organ rejection), cancer, or malnutrition are referred to as *acquired immunodeficiencies*.

Congenital B Cell Deficiencies

Examples of congenital B cell deficiencies include X-linked agammaglobulinemia and selective immunoglobulin isotype deficiencies, particularly IgG, IgA, and IgM. X-linked agammaglobulinemia is characterized by the absence of gamma globulin in the blood and is inherited as an X chromosome–linked disease. Affected males are susceptible to bacterial and some viral infections, but their frequency and severity can be reduced by periodic passive immunizations with pooled gamma globulin preparations. Afflicted individuals can and do respond to infections by most intracellular microbes and fungi, because these agents are eliminated primarily by immune T cells.

Congenital T Cell Deficiencies

Individuals with congenital T cell deficiencies exhibit increased susceptibility to infections with viruses, fungi, intracellular bacteria, and protozoa. These microorganisms are often capable of surviving and replicating inside cells, which is why their eradication is dependent on T cell immunity. Examples include DiGeorge syndrome (thymic hypoplasia—equivalent animal models include the nude mouse and rat) and types I and II bare lymphocyte syndrome. In the latter syndrome, there is a congenital underexpression of class II MHC molecules on APCs and B cells. Because these molecules are critically important in T cell activation, their absence results in an impairment of T cell function.

Combined Congenital T and B Cell Deficiencies

Severe combined immunodeficiency (SCID) refers to a heterogeneous group of disorders characterized by defective development of B and T cells. Several defects have been shown to independently result in the development of this condition. One type of SCID results from a deficiency of an enzyme called *adenosine deaminase* (ADA). This enzyme is required for the normal metabolism of the purine, adenosine, in lymphocytes, the absence of which results in the accumulation of toxic metabolites that destroy the cell. Attempts have been under way since 1990 to develop a way of transferring the gene for ADA into bone marrow cells from affected individuals as a means of restoring ADA production. Such gene transfer is carried out by a procedure referred to as *transfection* in which the gene is linked to the nucleic acid from a nonpathogenic virus that facilitates its entry into the host genome. This procedure is referred to as *gene therapy*. Although some of these patients have improved, the results are difficult to interpret because they also received synthetic ADA injections. Parenthetically, attempts at gene therapy have also been made for the treatment of hemophilia, cystic fibrosis, Gaucher's disease, alpha$_1$-antitrypsin deficiency (in emphysema), hemoglobinopathies, and familial hypercholesterolemia, as well as for several acquired, nongenetic diseases.[7]

SCID also develops as a result of a defect in the genes (called RAG-1 and RAG-2) that are responsible for the rearrangement and expression of antigen-receptor molecules. Finally, there are SCID cases that are X-linked that are a result of defects in the expression of a protein chain (γ) that is common to the receptors for IL-2, -4, -7, -9, and -15. Clearly, cells that are unable to respond to these cytokines suffer greatly in their ability to become activated by antigenic stimulation.

Congenital Defects Affecting Phagocytic Cells

Chronic granulomatous disease is a rare defect in macrophage and neutrophil function that results from a defect in the production of superoxide anion that is necessary for the destruction of phagocytosed bacteria. This defect initially results in the formation of numerous granulomas representing areas of fibrosis surrounded by a region of persistent intracellular infection. The disease is often fatal, even with intensive antibiotic therapy.

Acquired Immunodeficiency Syndrome

AIDS results from infection with one of two types of HIV viruses, HIV-1 or HIV-2. These viruses are referred to as *retroviruses* to indicate that they are RNA viruses that undergo reverse transcription to form DNA before their incorporation into the host genome. Other examples of retroviruses include HTLV-I and -II, which are associated with human adult T cell leukemia, and a host of other mammalian, avian, and reptilian viruses. The first confirmed cases of HIV infection were reported in 1981, though retrospective analysis revealed that a patient who died of unknown causes in 1959 was in fact infected with the AIDS virus.[8] Characterization of the virus began in 1985 when it was first isolated. To date, the World Health Organization estimates that more than 3 million adults and children have developed AIDS worldwide, and an additional 20 million are believed to be infected.

HIV is transmitted through sexual contact, parenteral exposure to blood products, and perinatal transmission during pregnancy or during the postpartum period. The populations most susceptible to HIV infection (HIV-1) are homosexual and bisexual men having unprotected sex, intravenous drug users, hemophiliacs receiving contaminated blood products, and infants of infected mothers—though increasing numbers of heterosexuals having unprotected sex are becoming infected. In many areas on the African continent, HIV sexual transmission (primarily HIV-2) appears to be primarily through heterosexual intercourse.

Clinical Features

Initial infection with HIV induces a potent immune response that is characterized by the development of fever, night sweats, joint pain, and lymphadenopathy in many patients. Others may not experience symptoms. These symptoms may appear weeks before the most commonly used blood test (which relies on the formation of anti-HIV antibodies) confirms the diagnosis of HIV infection. This is followed by a relatively long clinical latency period during which patients are symptom-free but the virus continues to replicate and lyse immune cells. When the immune system becomes compromised beyond a certain point, patients become susceptible to opportunistic infections, that is, infection by organisms that the immune system can no longer control. Some patients will experience night sweats, fevers, weight loss, generalized lymphadenopathy, diarrhea, and inflammatory skin conditions, collectively referred to as AIDS-related complex, or ARC. Full-blown AIDS follows, with patients experiencing opportunistic infections by organisms such as *Pneumocystis carinii, Candida, Mycobacterium tuberculosis,* and *Toxoplasma.* Other manifestations include the development of neoplasms such as Kaposi's sarcoma (a tumor of endothelial cells caused by herpes simplex virus), cachexia (progressive weight loss and diarrhea), encephalopathy, and numerous ocular manifestations that are discussed below.

Ocular Manifestations

The most commonly observed ophthalmologic abnormality in AIDS is cotton-wool spots, which are whitish, superficial, flocculent retinal blotches seen on fundoscopic examination. Histopathologically, these spots represent axonal swellings called *cytoid bodies* in the nerve fiber layer (Color Plate I). They are also seen in hypertension, diabetes, and lupus, and represent regions where there is an underlying disturbance in retinal microcirculation leading to areas of focal ischemic injury.[9]

The second most common ocular consequence of AIDS is CMV retinitis, which is seen in up to 40% of patients. On funduscopic examination,

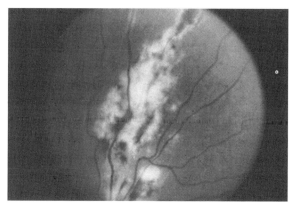

FIGURE 1.9. Areas of cytomegalovirus retinitis appear as well-demarcated, yellowish, flat lesions along the vascular arcades beginning at the posterior pole, often resulting in a wedge-shaped zone of retinal infection. (Reprinted with permission from E Ai. Cytomegalovirus Retinitis. In E Ai, I Ahmed [eds], AIDS and Ophthalmology: New Solutions. Ophthalmology Clinics of North America. Philadelphia: Saunders, 1997.)

CMV retinitis appears as well-demarcated, yellowish, flat lesions along the vascular arcades beginning at the posterior pole (Figure 1.9). Foci of hemorrhages are also seen. Retinal Müller cells and neurons can harbor the virus. Oral ganciclovir has been found to be safe and effective as maintenance therapy for CMV retinitis. Other treatments include the injection of ganciclovir or foscarnet intravitreously and the use of intraocular sustained-release implants.[10]

Other ophthalmic complications of HIV infection include Kaposi's sarcoma, ocular lymphoma, and molluscum contagiosum affecting the ocular adnexae, ophthalmic herpes zoster, corneal microsporidiosis, keratoconjunctivitis sicca, toxoplasmosis, and *P. carinii* choroiditis.[9]

Mechanism of Human Immunodeficiency Virus Infection

HIV consists of two identical strands of RNA encoding the genes for the viral envelope and core proteins, proteases, endonucleases, and reverse transcriptase, among others. The viral genome is encased within two layers of core proteins consisting of an inner capsid containing p24 proteins and an outer matrix consisting of p17 proteins. All the above are contained within an outer lipid bilayer consisting of numerous envelope proteins, including gp120 (glycoprotein of 120 kD) and gp41, which are cleaved from a common precursor protein called gp160 (Color Plate II).

The first step in HIV infection of a T helper cell or macrophage is the binding of the viral protein gp120 to the CD4 molecule on the surface of

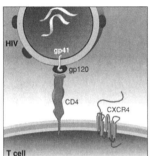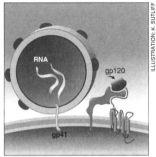

FIGURE 1.10.   After binding to CD4 on the surface of the T cell, HIV's gp120 binds to chemokine receptors such as CXCR4, allowing gp41 to breach the cell membrane. (HIV = human immunodeficiency virus.) (Reprinted with permission from J Cohen. Investigators detail HIV's fatal handshake. Science 1996;274:502. Copyright 1996, American Association for the Advancement of Science.)

the cell. This is followed by a conformational change resulting in the additional binding of gp120 to another molecule on the cell surface originally called *fusin*. This molecule, now called *CXCR4*, normally functions as a type of receptor for the chemokines RANTES, MIP-α, and MIP-1β. The importance of chemokine receptors in HIV infection was demonstrated by Gallo, Lusso, and their colleagues, who reported in 1995 that chemokines had the ability to protect cells from HIV infection.[11] In addition to CXCR4, two other chemokine receptors that are thought to play a role in HIV infection are CCR5 and CCR3. Evidence suggests that these receptors play a role in the infection of macrophages and some T cells, whereas the CXCR4 receptor plays a role in the infection of the majority of T cells. Interestingly, some individuals who are resistant to infection were shown to have mutations in their chemokine receptors.[12]

The conformational change that results from the binding of gp120 to a chemokine receptor facilitates the attachment of gp41 to the target cell surface and initiates the transfer of the HIV virion into the cell (Figure 1.10). The viral genome is then converted by viral reverse transcriptase into DNA, which then enters the host nucleus. Once in the nucleus, viral integrase catalyzes the incorporation of viral DNA, then called a provirus, into the host genome. The virus may lie dormant for varying amounts of time, becoming activated only upon specific activation of the target cell in response to antigenic- and cytokine-mediated stimulation. It has been shown that even in patients with normal lymphocyte numbers and stable peripheral blood virus titers, there is a terrible battle raging in the lymph nodes and spleen with the immune system working feverishly to produce new CD4+ cells to keep pace with HIV-mediated T cell destruction. The HIV-infected T cell dies when its incorporated viral DNA begins to produce (i.e., transcribe) mature viral particles. Under the influence of viral protease enzymes, the newly generated viral RNA is packaged into virions that are then released from the dying cell and attack neighboring cells.

Immune System Response to Human
Immunodeficiency Virus Infection

The most important immunologic consequence of HIV infection is the direct lysis of disease-fighting CD4+ T cells and macrophages. However, until such time that profound immunosuppression occurs as a result of T cell depletion, the immune system wages a formidable battle against the virus, using both antibodies and cellular immune mediators. The formation of antibodies in newly infected individuals takes several weeks to develop and is the basis of the available screening tests. As with many pathogenic organisms, HIV has developed ways of evading immune detection, including viral mutation. Another mechanism involves the expression of the HIV *nef* protein. Expression of this protein by the virus has been associated with a downregulation of MHC class I molecules from the infected cell's surface, resulting in a reduced capacity of the cell to stimulate cytotoxic T cell mediated lysis.[13]

Therapeutic Approach to Acquired
Immunodeficiency Syndrome

Azidothymidine (AZT), a reverse transcriptase inhibitor, was the first AIDS drug to be developed. It slowed the progression of AIDS but, at least in some patients, accelerated the time to death once symptoms developed. More recently, it was shown to play an important role in reducing the transmission of virus from an infected mother to her unborn child. Other reverse transcriptase inhibitors include dideoxyinosine and dideoxycytidine. Newer agents inhibit the proteases required for the packaging of new virions for release from the infected cell. These protease inhibitors are now being used in conjunction with two different types of reverse transcriptase inhibitors in a cocktail referred to as *triple therapy*. This approach has been very effective in significantly reducing viral load and has accounted for the fact that the number of deaths due to AIDS has recently gone down. The concern with all of these agents is that the mutated forms of the enzymes that they inhibit become drug resistant; this phenomenon has been attributed to AZT's loss of effectiveness when used alone. What role chemokines may play in future treatment strategies designed to block viral attachment remains to be explored.

Background Material

Text sources for background material include I Roitt, J Brostoff, D Male. Immunology (4th ed). London: Mosby, 1996; and AK Abbas, AH Lichtman, JS Pober. Cellular and Molecular Immunology (3rd ed). Philadelphia: Saunders, 1997.

References

1. Danesh J, Collins R, Appleby P, Peto R. Association of fibrinogen C-reactive protein, albumin, or leukocyte count with coronary heart disease: meta analysis of prospective studies. JAMA 1998;279:1477–1482.
2. Grau GE, Maenel DN. TNF inhibition and sepsis—sounding a cautionary note. Nat Med 1997;3:1193–1195.
3. White SH, Wimley WC, Selsted ME. Structure, function, and membrane integration of defensins. Curr Opin Struct Biol 1995;5:521–527.
4. Ganz T, Lehrer RI. Defensins. Pharmacol Ther 1995;66:191–205.
5. Tam EK, Caughey GH. Degradation of airway neuropeptides by human lung tryptase. Am J Respir Cell Mol Biol 1990;3:27–32.
6. Roitt I, Brostoff J, Male D. Immunology (4th ed). London: Mosby, 1996;8–9.
7. Verma I, Somia N. Gene therapy—promises, problems, and prospects. Nature 1997;389:239–242.
8. Zhu T, Korber BT, Nahamias AJ, et al. An African HIV-1 sequence from 1959 and implications for the origin of the epidemic. Nature 1998;391:594–596.
9. Ah-Fat FG, Batterbury M. Ophthalmic complications of HIV/AIDS. Postgrad Med J 1996;72:725–730.
10. Musch D, Martin DF, Gordon JF, et al. Treatment of cytomegalovirus retinitis with a sustained-release ganciclovir implant. N Engl J Med 1997;337:83–90.
11. Cocchi F, DeVico AL, Garzino-Demo A, et al. Identification of RANTES, MIP-1 alpha, and MIP-1 beta as the major HIV-suppressive factors produced by CD8+ T cells. Science 1995;270:1811–1815.
12. Dean M, Carrington M, Winkler C, et al. Genetic restriction of HIV-1 infection and progression to AIDS by a deletion allele of the CKR5 structural gene. Science 1996;273:1856–1862.
13. Collins KL, Chen BK, Kalams SA, et al. HIV-1 Nef protein protects infected primary cells against killing by cytotoxic T lymphocytes. Nature 1998;391:397–401.

CHAPTER 2

Ocular Immune Privilege

Privilege: a right or immunity granted as a peculiar benefit, advantage, or favor

When donor tissues or organs are transplanted across a histocompatibility barrier, an immune response is initiated in the recipient that ultimately results in the graft's destruction. It has been known for more than a century, however, that particular regions of the body afford protection to such grafts, allowing them to survive for prolonged periods.[1,2] These sites are referred to as being *immunologically privileged*[3] and include such diverse regions as the placenta, testis (Figure 2.1), brain, hair follicle, hamster cheek pouch, liver, peritoneal omental pouch, mature cartilage, ovary, thyroid, and the retina, iris, ciliary body, anterior chamber, cornea, lens, and vitreous cavity of the eye.[3–5] Long-term survival of a tissue or organ allograft can occur in a host if the graft itself is nonimmunogenic; the graft is sequestered from the immune system; or effector immune mechanisms capable of destroying the graft are inhibited.

It is important to note at the outset that although immune privilege was initially described as a site's unique inability to reject transplanted tissues, it has come to refer in more general terms to a region in which all, or some elements of, the normal immune response to a host of antigens are lacking.

Factors Contributing to Immune Privilege

Graft Immunogenicity

The immunogenicity of a graft is determined by the presence of cell surface allogeneic major histocompatibility complex (MHC) molecules, which are recognized by the host by the indirect or direct pathway described in the previous chapter. Graft immunogenicity can be reduced by masking

43

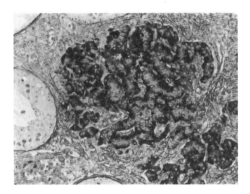

FIGURE 2.1.   Photomicrograph of a xenograft of rat islets of Langerhans in the testis of a diabetic mouse 60 days after transplantation. The islets were stained with aldehyde fuchsin, which revealed well-granulated cells. (Reprinted with permission from B Bobzien, Y Yasunami, M Majercik, et al. Intratesticular transplants of islet xenografts [rat to mouse]. Diabetes 1983;32:213–216.)

MHC molecules through the use of monoclonal antibodies or eliminating them by transgenic means, or by removal of class II+ passenger leukocytes from the graft. However, transplantations into privileged sites have used unmanipulated, immunogenic grafts without adverse immune consequence. Consequently, enhanced graft survival in privileged sites cannot be attributed to changes in graft immunogenicity.

Immunologic Isolation

Immune privilege has been theorized to result from the absence of either a vasculature or a draining lymphatic system in the privileged site, from the presence of a vascular barrier, or from the absence or aberrant function of MHC molecules.

Absence of a Vascular Supply

Examples of privileged sites that lack a blood supply are cartilage, the lens, and the cornea (not the corneal limbus, which is vascularized). These tissues meet their nutritional requirements in different ways. In cartilage, the chondrocytes receive nutrients and oxygen by diffusion through the cartilage matrix from vessels located outside the perichondrium. The lens receives some oxygen from the aqueous humor which is used primarily by its epithelium and cortex. Most of the carbohydrate usage by the lens is by way of anaerobic metabolism. In the cornea, oxygen in the ambient air readily diffuses into the epithelium and most of the stroma, whereas the corneal endothelium probably receives its oxygen from the aqueous humor.[6] Carbon dioxide produced in all levels of the cornea appears to dif-

TABLE 2.1
Elements of the Blood-Ocular Barrier

Thick, fibrous, acellular connective tissue surrounding iris vasculature
Ciliary body epithelial cells linked by junctional complexes
Retinal pigment epithelial cells linked by junctional complexes
Retinal endothelial cells linked by tight junctions
Reduced endocytic vesicles in pigment epithelium and retinal endothelium

---

fuse outward. Parenthetically, in spite of the lack of a vascular supply, cartilage allografts are still susceptible to rejection apparently because chondrocytes themselves are highly immunogenic.[7]

Vascularization of a previously nonvascularized privileged site, such as the central cornea, correlates highly with its rejection following transplantation.[8] As we will see, other factors such as the presence of suppressor factors in aqueous humor also contribute to corneal immune privilege.

Presence of a Vascular Barrier

In vascularized immunologically privileged sites such as the brain, iris, ciliary body, and retina, the entry of immunologic effectors is blocked by specialized endothelial intercellular junctions. In the iris, ciliary body, and retina, these specializations are referred to as the *blood-ocular barrier*. This barrier limits the intraocular movement of immune cells such as granulocytes, lymphocytes, and monocytes and factors such as certain plasma proteins, including complement components and alpha$_2$-macroglobulin, a protease inhibitor.[9] Thus, immune reactions are prevented by exclusion. Interestingly, as articulated by Streilein,[10] because some of these factors can act to both promote and suppress immunogenic inflammation, the eye consequently lacks the ability to regulate ocular inflammation.

The specific elements that contribute to the blood-ocular barrier (Table 2.1) differ in different regions of the eye. In the iris, vessels are enclosed in a thick, fibrous, acellular connective tissue. In the ciliary body, the cells of the two epithelial layers are joined together by junctional complexes which serve a dual purpose. First, they transmit the movement of the ciliary muscle to the inner layer, and second, they serve as a barrier between the blood and the intraocular environment. The retinal pigment epithelial cells are interconnected by a junctional complex consisting of apical gap junctions, tight junctions, and a zonula adherens. The retinal outer plexiform and outer nuclear layers, and the fovea, are vessel-free zones, and the endothelial cells of all other retinal vessels are linked by tight junctions. Finally, both the pigment epithelial cells and retinal endothelial cells have a paucity of endocytic vesicles and tightly regulate their ionic and metabolic gradients.[11]

Although morphologic evidence of the existence of a blood-ocular barrier has been amply reported, a study by Prendergast et al.[12] has questioned its physiologic existence. These authors used fluorescent labeling to track the distribution of activated T cell blasts in the retina. Their results showed that labeled cells freely entered and exited the retina but only remained there if they were activated and were responding to retinal antigens as in uveoretinitis. In this latter case, there was ultimately a progressive inflammatory disruption of the barrier, resulting in more pronounced leukocyte infiltration and edema. If their study can be confirmed, it will open debate about the immunologic significance of all tight junction–mediated barriers.

Role of Lymphatics

For many years after its initial description, immune privilege was thought to be a result of the absence of a lymphatic drainage in the privileged site. Lymphatic vessels channel antigens to draining lymph nodes that trap them in their cortex and facilitate their binding to appropriate antigen-presenting cells (APCs) and lymphocytes, initiating an immune response. Removal of a draining lymph node prior to transplantation into the region of a skin allograft prevents rejection.[13] It was theorized that if antigens placed into privileged sites did not have access to draining lymph nodes, they would be effectively concealed from the immune system.

Although certain immune privileged sites, such as the hamster cheek pouch, do in fact lack a lymphatic drainage,[14] others have indeed been shown to possess such vessels or to otherwise have access to draining nodes. For example, the testis has been shown to possess two distinct lymphatic spaces that drain fluid at different rates.[15] Some of these lymphatic vessels are quite long, a fact that has been used to explain testicular immune privilege.[16] In the brain, fluid enters the tissue by slow permeation across cerebral capillaries and eventually flows out into the cerebrospinal fluid (CSF). CSF, in turn, drains into venous blood by a mechanism involving passive hydrostatic pressurization across arachnoid villi situated in the walls of dural sinuses. Although this pathway accounts for most of the CSF drainage, a small amount takes another route that ultimately transports it to cervical lymph nodes. Sleeves of subarachnoid CSF surround a portion of various cranial and spinal nerves, in particular, the olfactory and optic nerves. Under the influence of a positive pressure gradient, the CSF makes it way through these nerves into the submucosal tissue of the eye and nose, regions that drain by lymphatic vessels into cervical nodes (Figure 2.2).[17]

By far, the bulk of the aqueous humor, like CSF, drains directly into the vasculature, in this case by way of the canal of Schlemm. Drainage of intraocular fluid into lymph nodes has been shown to occur, however, in ways analogous to that described above for CSF. Lymphatic drainage of the intraocular environment occurs via the uveoscleral pathway (Figure 2.3).[18] It has been

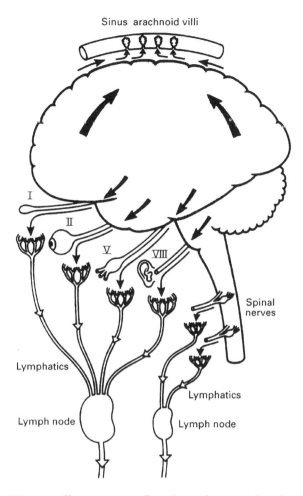

Sinus arachnoid villi

Spinal
nerves

Lymphatics

Lymphatics

Lymph node

Lymph node

FIGURE 2.2. Diagram illustrating outflow from the cranial and spinal subarachnoid spaces along two pathways: across arachnoid villi into sinus blood, and along certain cranial and spinal nerves into cervical lymphatic vessels. (Reprinted with permission from PM Knopf, HF Cserr, SC Nolan, et al. Physiology and immunology of lymphatic drainage of interstitial and cerebrospinal fluid from the brain. Neuropathol Appl Neurobiol 1995;21:175–180.)

estimated that approximately 10% of the aqueous humor drains by this mechanism into lymphatic vessels in the head and neck.[10] What role the uveoscleral pathway may have in ocular immunity remains to be elucidated.

Role of Antigen-Presenting Cells and Major Histocompatibility Complex Antigen Expression

Bone marrow–derived APCs, characterized by their expression of class II MHC molecules, play a critical role in the initiation and propagation of an

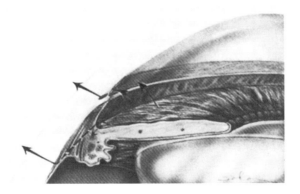

FIGURE 2.3.   Two principal pathways of aqueous flow: trabeculocanalicular (top) and uveoscleral (bottom). (Reprinted with permission from WM Hart [ed], Adler's Physiology of the Eye—Clinical Application [9th ed]. St. Louis: Mosby–Year Book, 1992;254.)

immune response. These cells pick up antigens that enter tissues and migrate to a draining lymph node where they present them to T cells. This process leads to T cell activation and to the generation of lymphocyte effector cells and factors. APCs can also activate lymphocytes within a tissue itself. It follows that if a tissue or organ lacks APCs, it might be far less likely to promulgate an antigen-specific immune response. Thus, the localized absence or reduction in number of APCs could play a role in mediating immune privilege.

Class II molecules have been shown to be inducible on cells not classically thought of as APCs. The presence of these molecules on otherwise nonimmune cells has in some cases been shown to afford the cells the capacity to present antigen to T cells. However, not all such class II+ cells have demonstrated an ability to initiate an antigen-specific immune response; some have even been shown to suppress immune reactivity.

Cytotoxic T cells are immunologically restricted to class I molecules, which are present on most body cells. It follows that if cells lack class I expression, they would be less susceptible to the lytic action of cytotoxic T cells. This is yet another mechanism that can contribute to immune privilege.

Placenta.   The placenta expresses a unique class I molecule called HLA-G,[19] which is only expressed in one other tissue, the fetal eye.[20] The placenta also lacks class II expression.[21] Interestingly, the expression of placental class II has been linked to the occurrence of miscarriages.[21]

Brain.   The brain normally expresses very low levels of MHC class I and II molecules. However, many different cell types in the brain can be induced to express these molecules. Class I is inducible on electrically silent, presumably impaired, neurons by interferon-gamma (IFN-γ); this restricted activation may play a role in promoting cytotoxic T cell removal of these neurons.[22] IFN-γ also induces class II expression on astrocytes, microglia, endothelial cells, and smooth muscle/pericyte cells. Many of these cells have been shown to have the capacity to present myelin-derived peptides and play an important role in the development of central nervous system inflammation, such as in the case of encephalomyelitis.[23] Thus, although brain tissue is immunologically silent vis-à-vis antigen presentation under normal conditions, it has the potential under the influence of soluble immune mediators to become immunologically active.

This evidence notwithstanding, immune privileged sites do not always lack class II+ APCs, nor do they fail to express class I antigens. Two examples of this are the testis and the eye. All cells in the mature testis have been shown to express class I antigens, and numerous class II+ cells were demonstrated in the testicular interstitium.[24] A description of the class I antigen and class II cell distribution in the eye follows.

Eye. Immunohistochemical and flow-cytometric techniques revealed that class I antigen is constitutively expressed on cells of the trabecular meshwork and corneal endothelium, stroma, and epithelium,[7,25,26] as well as on the pigmented and nonpigmented cells of the ciliary body, the anterior border of the iris, the vascular endothelium of the uvea,[27] and retinal pigment epithelial cells.[28] Expression was generally submaximal, particularly in the cornea. Because cytotoxic T cells recognize viral antigen in conjunction with class I molecules on the surface of infected cells, their reduced level in the cornea could conceivably contribute to persistence of a viral pathogen in this tissue. On the other hand, corneal class I expression can be upregulated by numerous inflammatory cytokines, in particular IFN-γ.[28] It is noteworthy that lens epithelial cells do not normally express class I,[29] a fact that, together with the presence of a lens capsule and the absence of a vascular supply, contributes to its immune privilege.

It has been clearly demonstrated that the central cornea is devoid of class II+ Langerhans' cells.[30] However, the corneal limbus contains these cells which, in response to infectious agents,[31] chemical irritants,[32] or localized damage,[33] migrate into the central cornea. The presence of Langerhans' cells in the central cornea was shown not only to facilitate inflammation, but also to interfere with unique immunosuppressive features of the anterior chamber,[34] as described later.

For many years, there have been conflicting reports concerning the presence of class II+ cells in the iris and ciliary body. Resolution of this controversy began in the late 1980s with the introduction of better methods for the preparation of iris and ciliary body tissues. Using these methods, it was reported that the iris and ciliary body of rodents contained a significant number of cells of bone marrow origin, some of which

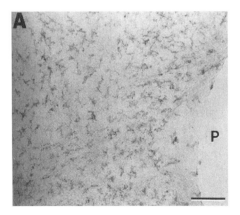
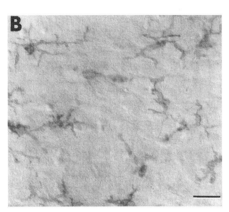

FIGURE 2.4.   Low (A) and medium (B) magnification light micrographs of stained class II+ cells in the murine iris. Note the classic dendritic morphology of these cells. (P = pupil; bar in A = 500 mm; bar in B = 100 mm.) (Reprinted with permission from TL Knisely, TM Anderson, ME Sherwood, et al. Morphologic and ultrastructural examination of I-A+ cells in the murine iris. Invest Ophthalmol Vis Sci 1991;32:2423–2431. Copyright 1991, Association for Research in Vision and Ophthalmology.)

expressed class II molecules and most of which expressed the macrophage marker F4/80.[35] Ultrastructurally, these cells were shown to resemble classic antigen-presenting dendritic cells[36] and to reside between the two epithelial cell layers of the ciliary epithelium and beneath the single layer of the epithelium of the iris (Figure 2.4).[37] Classic macrophages were also shown to be present. Similarly, confocal microscopy revealed a regular array of macrophages and class II+ dendritic cells in the human iris.[38]

Other intraocular regions that were shown to possess class II+ dendritic cells were the trabecular meshwork (but not in the direct outflow pathway) and along the uveoscleral pathway,[39] as well as near the ora serrata.[37] In humans, ramified retinal microglial cells were shown to have features in common with dendritic cells, including the constitutive expression of class II,[40] whereas rat retinal microglia lack class II.[37] Müller cells, though not constitutive expressors of class II molecules, can be induced to express them.[41] Macrophages were also found throughout intraocular tissues. Although the choroid lies outside the blood-ocular barrier, it is important to note the existence of dendritic cells in the connective tissues surrounding the choriocapillaris and choroid, because they play a role in ocular inflammation.

Although they express class II, iris and ciliary body cells do not act as professional APCs. They are unable to present alloantigens to T cells and, in fact, suppress mixed lymphocyte reactions when they are added as regulatory cells.[35,42] Even treatment with subinflammatory doses of IFN-γ fails to promote immunogenic antigen presentation by these cells. Similar results were obtained using suspensions of murine Müller cells, which failed to activate retinal S-antigen (S-Ag)–specific T cell lines.[41] Only after culture in granulocyte-macrophage colony-stimulating factor (GM-CSF) did dendritic cells from the iris display stimulating ability on par with Langerhans' cells taken from the skin.[42] Cells obtained from the corneal limbus, however, were allostimulatory.

Thus, even though cells with the appearance of classic APCs are present in the immune privileged regions of the eye, they fail to activate immunity. A great deal of data attribute this fact to the influence of factors, present in the aqueous humor, on these cells. Not only do these factors, discussed below, affect class II+ cells in the eye, but they also directly suppress lymphocyte activity and as such contribute on two levels to ocular immune privilege.

Suppression of Effector Immune Mechanisms

Immunosuppressive Factors in the Eye

It was first demonstrated in the early 1970s that aqueous humor suppresses lymphocyte proliferation.[43] Later it was shown more specifically that aqueous humor inhibited mixed lymphocyte reactions and cytokine production in response to MHC alloantigens, soluble antigens, and interleukin-2 (IL-2)–dependent T cell proliferation.[44] A notable exception to the immunosuppressive nature of aqueous humor was that it did not inhibit fully differentiated cytotoxic T cells from binding to and lysing target cells.

The absence of certain plasma proteins, such as many of the complement proteins and cortisol-binding globulin (CBG), undoubtedly contributes to the immunosuppressiveness of aqueous humor (interestingly, many are increased in inflamed eyes as a compensatory mechanism). Aqueous humor contains low levels of IgG but other immunoglobulin isotypes are absent. However, it is becoming clear that it is not the absence of immune activators but the presence of immunosuppressive factors that contributes to the immunoinhibitory nature of the intraocular environment (Table 2.2). These include vasoactive intestinal polypeptide (VIP), alpha–melanocyte stimulating hormone (α-MSH), calcitonin gene-related protein (CGRP), cortisol, and transforming growth factor–beta (TGF-β).[45]

Vasoactive Intestinal Polypeptide. VIP suppresses lymphocyte proliferation under various stimulatory conditions, seemingly by inhibiting IL-2 production, and regulates the migratory activity of T cells.[46,47] In contrast, VIP stimulates immunoglobulin production by, and the growth of, B cells.[48] In addition to its presence in aqueous humor, VIP immunoreactivity has been localized in nerve fibers in the choroid and anterior and posterior uvea,[49] suggesting that they may be the source of aqueous humor VIP.

Alpha–Melanocyte Stimulating Hormone. α-MSH suppresses IFN-γ production but does not affect lymphocyte proliferation.[50] It may also antagonize the proinflammatory effects of interleukin-1 (IL-1) and TNF-α.[51]

TABLE 2.2
Immunosuppressive Factors in Aqueous Humor

Transforming growth factor–beta
Vasoactive intestinal polypeptide
Alpha–melanocyte stimulating hormone
Calcitonin gene-related peptide
Cortisol
Natural killer cell inhibitory factor (10 kD)

Calcitonin Gene-Related Protein.   CGRP inhibits delayed-type hypersensitivity (DTH).[52] Like VIP, CGRP has also been localized in ocular nerves, specifically in sensory nerves in the anterior uvea. CGRP released from these nerves has been shown to mediate hyperemia in the anterior segment, increased intraocular pressure, breakdown of the blood-aqueous barrier, and the induction of miosis.[53] Evidence suggests that these nerves are the source of CGRP in the aqueous humor.

Cortisol.   Cortisol, which is known to have immunosuppressive effects, has been shown to be present in aqueous humor in concentrations similar to that in the blood. In serum, cortisol is bound to the globulin CBG, or transcortin. Bound cortisol appears to be physiologically inactive. CBG has been shown to be absent from aqueous humor.[54] It is therefore likely that cortisol in aqueous humor acts as an immunosuppressive factor.

Natural Killer Cell Inhibitory Factor.   Aqueous humor was also shown to contain a factor with an approximate molecular weight of 10 kD, which inhibits natural killer (NK) cell activity.[55] NK cells recognize target cells that have reduced expression of class I on their cell surface, particularly tumor cells. Corneal endothelial cells also have reduced expression of class I. It was theorized that this factor might be important in protecting corneal endothelial cells from unprovoked attack by NK cells (Table 2.2).

Transforming Growth Factor–Beta

Multiple Tissue Effects.   Although the above factors unquestionably play a role in suppressing immune reactions in the anterior chamber, many of the inhibitory effects of aqueous humor can be attributed to TGF-β. This cytokine was originally characterized as a factor capable of promoting the anchorage-independent growth of nontransformed rat fibroblasts in soft agar medium,[56] but it has become increasingly clear that it has diverse biological effects and is produced by many different cell types. It inhibits the growth of most epithelial cells[57] and stimulates the growth of some fibroblasts, osteoblasts, and Schwann cells.[58] Myogenesis, adipogenesis, and hematopoiesis are inhibited by TGF-β; osteogenesis and chondrogenesis are promoted.[59] TGF-β stimulates the formation of connective tissue matrix molecules such as collagen, fibronectin, tenascin (embryonic mes-enchymal protein), glycosaminoglycans, osteonectin, osteospondin, and thrombospondin,[60] and plays an important role in wound healing.

Immune Effects. TGF-β also plays a role in immune regulation and is pro-duced by macrophages, monocytes, and B and T lymphocytes.[61] Exogenous TGF-β inhibits T lymphocyte and thymocyte proliferation,[62,63] IL-2 receptor expression,[64] B cell proliferation and immunoglobulin production,[65] the devel opment of cytotoxic T lymphocytes,[66,67] the generation of lymphokine-acti-vated killer (LAK) cells, the generation and activity of NK cells,[68] and class II expression on tumor cells.[69] It is noteworthy that many of these effects are reversible with cytokines such as tumor necrosis factor (TNF), IFN-γ, and IL-1. For example, in contrast to TGF-β, TNF enhances cytotoxic T cell develop-ment, IL-2 receptor expression, class II antigen expression, interferon produc-tion, NK activity, thymocyte proliferation, and B cell proliferation.[68]

The bifunctional nature of TGF-β, described above in relation to its opposing effects on cell proliferation in various tissues, is also manifested in its role as an immune regulator. For example, though TGF-β generally reduces immunoglobulin (Ig) production, it increases the secretion of IgA. Although it inhibits NK activity, it downregulates class I expression on tumor cells, rendering them susceptible to lysis by NK cells that recognize cells that are missing such molecules. It also does not block the activity of cytotoxic T cells. These effects have implications for ocular immunity. TGF-β is present in tears where it likely plays a role in suppressing ocular surface inflammation, promoting normal growth and differentiation of ocular surface epithelia, and promoting wound healing.[70] Tears also con-tain IgA, secretion of which is increased by TGF-β, as mentioned above.

Three isoforms of TGF-β, each a 25-kD homodimer, exist in mam-mals: TGF-β1, -β2, and -β3. Each of these molecules is secreted as biologi-cally inactive complexes which can become activated on acidification, alkalinization, heating, treatment with urea,[71] or by the enzymatic action of plasmin[72,73] or sialidase.[74]

Transforming Growth Factor–Beta in the Eye. TGF-β, predominantly the TGF-β2 isoform, was shown to be present in normal aqueous humor in several different species including humans[75–77] in immunosuppressive concentrations (Table 2.3). The source of aqueous TGF-β was established to be the ciliary epithelial cells.[78,79] Interestingly, the levels of TGF-β2 in aqueous humor were reduced in cases of ocular inflammation such as uveitis.[80] TGF-β1 and/or TGF-β2 are also produced by a host of other intraocular cells and tissues in the human and primate eye, including retinal pigment epithelial cells,[81] the super-ficial limbal epithelial cells, conjunctival stroma, ciliary processes, and stroma adjacent to the pigment epithelium,[82] Müller cells, ganglion cells, photorecep-tors, hyalocytes, and cells associated with choroidal and retinal vessels.[83]

Plasmin is an activator of TGF-β. (It also activates collagenase and metalloproteinases.) Plasmin is formed from its inactive precursor, plas-

TABLE 2.3
Location of Transforming Growth Factor–Beta in the Eye

Ciliary epithelium and process
Retinal pigment epithelial cells
Corneal limbal epithelial cells
Conjunctival stroma
Stroma adjacent to pigment epithelium in the pars plana
Müller cells
Ganglion cells
Photoreceptors
Hyalocytes
Cells associated with choroidal and retinal vessels

minogen, by plasminogen activator, of which there are two types: tissue plasminogen activator (t-PA) and urokinase plasminogen activator (u-PA). This conversion is inhibited by plasminogen activation inhibitor–1 (PAI-1). Aqueous humor contains significant amounts of plasminogen and t-PA,[84,85] but only traces of PAI-1. Intraocular t-PA appears to be derived from the choroid.[86] Although it is likely that the presence of t-PA and the low levels of its inhibitor help to keep the aqueous outflow pathways patent, they may also play a role in the activation of intraocular TGF-β and in matrix remodeling in the tissues lining the anterior and posterior chambers. Parenthetically, TGF-β has been shown to regulate the activity of t-PA in different tumor cells, including human uveal melanoma cells.[87]

Fas Ligand–Induced Apoptosis

In Chapter 1, Fas and Fas ligand (FasL) were discussed in relation to the regulation of the immune response. Binding of a lymphocyte that expresses Fas to FasL induces the programmed cell death, or apoptosis, of the Fas-containing cell. Elimination of activated T cells following eradication of antigen is thought to occur by such a mechanism.

FasL mRNA has been shown to be expressed in the eye.[88] Immunohistochemical analysis localized FasL on the corneal epithelium and endothelium, iris and ciliary body, and throughout the retina.[88,89] Intraocular FasL induced apoptosis in immune cells infiltrating into the anterior chamber following infection.[88] Apoptosis failed to occur, under similar conditions, in animals expressing the gene *gld* (generalized lymphoproliferative disease), which encodes a mutant, nonfunctional Fas.[90] (These animals display increased lymphocyte counts and develop an autoimmune disease similar to systemic lupus erythematosus [SLE].) Thus, the interaction of lymphocytes expressing Fas with FasL in the eye contributes to ocular immune privilege. Interestingly, a similar expression of FasL was also demonstrated in another privileged site, the testis.[91]

Many factors contribute to immune privilege in the eye and elsewhere. In a sense, though, the eye, and in particular its anterior chamber, is unique. The cells and factors in this region interact in a targeted way, providing the eye with the means to eliminate foreign antigens without sacrificing visual integrity. This specialized intraocular immune response is described below.

Role of Anterior Chamber–Associated Immune Deviation in Ocular Immunity

It was once observed that allogeneic lymphoid cells injected into the anterior chamber of the rat eye failed to elicit significant DTH inflammation.[92] This finding itself was not unexpected in light of what is currently known about the immunosuppressive nature of aqueous humor. What was interesting, however, was that recipient rats had an impaired ability to reject orthotopic skin allografts derived from the same donor as the lymphoid cells. Since its first description, this phenomenon has been elicited experimentally in animals using a wide variety of antigens such as bovine serum albumen (BSA),[93] ovalbumin,[94] retinal proteins,[95] hapten-derivatized cells,[96] virally encoded antigens (herpes simplex virus [HSV]),[97] alloantigens[98] (an intact B cell population was also shown to be necessary for the induction of this phenomenon), and tumor-specific antigens.[99,100] The stereotypic, altered systemic immune response to antigens placed in the anterior chamber is termed *anterior chamber–associated immune deviation* (ACAID).[101] The immune deviation that occurs in ACAID is characterized by impaired development and expression of antigen-specific DTH[102,103] and impaired production of complement-fixing antibodies (isotype IgG2a).[104] Elements of the immune response that are intact include the ability to produce noncomplement-fixing antibodies[104] and the cytotoxic T cell–mediated lysis of target cells (Table 2.4).[102]

As mentioned, TGF-β is present in abundance in aqueous humor and has immunosuppressive effects. However, it does not inhibit the activity of cytotoxic T cells and its effects on antibody production are variable. The term *immune deviation* was selected to describe ACAID because ACAID shares some of the features of the immune response to soluble antigens first described with this terminology.[105]

Enucleation of the eye up to 4 days, or removal of the spleen up to 6 days, after anterior chamber antigen injection aborted ACAID induction.[106,107] These observations gave rise to the concept that there was an immunologic link between the eye and the spleen that was important in

TABLE 2.4
Systemic Immune Alterations in Anterior Chamber–Associated
Immune Deviation

Suppressed	Delayed-type hypersensitivity reaction
	Production of complement-fixing antibodies (IgG2a)
Intact	Cytotoxic T cell activity
	Production of non–complement-fixing antibodies

this phenomenon. This link was referred to as the *camerosplenic axis*. It was reasoned that the ACAID-inducing signal, be it a soluble factor or cellular constituent, would travel from the eye to the spleen in the vasculature. Investigators reasoned that this "signal" would accumulate in the blood if the spleen were removed. This held true and led to the isolation of ACAID-inducing cells and factors.

Nature of the Anterior Chamber–Associated Immune Deviation–Inducing Signal

Using the above approach, it was shown that the ACAID-inducing signal was not antigenic itself. Furthermore, the signal was shown to be associated with either the serum component[108] or monocytes, as recognized by monoclonal antibody F4/80,[106] in the blood, depending on the nature of the antigen.[107] F4/80+ monocytes represent a significant population of MHC class II positive cells, of bone marrow origin, that are present in the eye. Although these cells appear to be classic APCs, they fail to stimulate allogeneic T cells.[35,42] F4/80+ cells harvested from eyes previously injected with BSA induced ACAID when injected into syngeneic recipients; F4/80+ cells harvested from the peritoneal cavity 24 hours after intraperitoneal (i.p.) injection of BSA did not. However, when peritoneal exudate cells (PECs) from naive mice were pulsed with BSA overnight in vitro and then injected into the anterior chamber of normal mice, the recipients developed ACAID.[93] These data suggested that the local microenvironment of the anterior chamber influenced the action of classic APCs, conferring on them ACAID-inducing properties. Specifically, it was shown that TGF-β in the aqueous humor was responsible for bestowing ACAID-inducing properties on these PECs.[109-111] In fact, culture of PECs, or peripheral blood monocytes,[112] along with antigen and TGF-β was shown to be sufficient to convert these cells into ACAID-inducers. Exogenous TGF-β was shown to have two effects on PECs: it enhanced the secretion of TGF-β by the PECs,[113] and it reduced the production of IL-12 and expression of CD40 by the PECs.[114] These effects were speculated to play a role in the inability of the PECs to promote the development of Th1 cells involved in the DTH response.[114]

Nature of the Final Immune Effector Cells That Suppress Delayed-Type Hypersensitivity

The effector mechanism of ACAID seems to differ depending on whether the animal was primed or unprimed to the antigen.[115,116] In unprimed animals, when PECs are cultured with antigen in the presence of TGF-β, the antigen is cleaved, and peptide fragments are preferentially incorporated into class I molecules on these cells, which probably accounts for the selective activation of CD8+ regulatory (suppressor) and cytotoxic cells in the spleens of animals with ACAID.[113] Thus, DTH responses and the development of precursors of cytotoxic T cells are inhibited, and the activity of cytotoxic T cells is promoted.

In primed animals or in animals in which T cells are injected along with antigen into the eye or the antigen (e.g., HSV) elicits inflammation that includes T cells,[115] it appears that a soluble ACAID-inducing factor is involved. Specifically, the soluble factor appears to resemble a chain of the T cell antigen receptor[117] that was either deposited or migrated into the eye.[115] It has been suggested that the binding of Fas+ T cells to FasL in the eye may promote the deposition of these chains in the anterior chamber.[115]

Role of Cytokines Other Than Transforming Growth Factor–Beta in Anterior Chamber–Associated Immune Deviation

Systemic administration of IL-1 or IL-2 interferes with ACAID induction; IL-1 presumably prevents ACAID by promoting IL-2 production.[118,119] Similarly, local production of IFN-γ, a potent inhibitor of TGF-β, prevents the induction of ACAID. Yet, TNF-α, IL-4, and IL-10 have been implicated in successful ACAID induction.[120,121,122,123]

Does Light Affect Anterior Chamber–Associated Immune Deviation?

The fact that ACAID occurs in the eye, an organ that has evolved to receive and transmit light images, led investigators to explore whether light itself might play a role in ACAID. The known effect of ultraviolet light in promoting suppressor cell development lent credence to this theory.[124] Injection of antigenic cells into the anterior chamber of dark-adapted eyes (>18 hours in darkness) evoked a conventional systemic immune response, that is, ACAID was prevented.[125] The demonstration that the intraocular levels of VIP fell and substance P rose in dark-adapted animals suggested that one or both of these factors might mediate this effect. This was supported by data showing that a VIP-receptor antagonist, when injected into the eye with antigen, reversed ACAID in daylight-adapted eyes, whereas a substance P receptor antagonist restored ACAID to dark-adapted eyes.[126]

It is also conceivable that changes in the uveoscleral outflow may play a role in the loss of ACAID in dark-adapted eyes. Contraction of the ciliary muscle is known to reduce the uveoscleral flow and its relaxation has the opposite effect. Increasing uveoscleral flow by topical application of prostaglandin $F_{2\text{-alpha}}$ ($PGF_{2\alpha}$) blocked ACAID.[127] Because there is a reduced level of accommodation at night, uveoscleral flow might be increased, resulting in antigenic drainage to cervical lymph nodes where a classic immune response can be initiated.

Clinical Significance of Anterior Chamber–Associated Immune Deviation

The eye, like other tissues and organs in the body, must possess the immunologic resources to rid itself of foreign invaders and transformed cells. The immune response that most effectively eliminates these antigens is the DTH reaction. Although the DTH reaction can occur without adverse consequences in most organs, this is not true of the eye. The cytoarchitectural organization of the neural retina is unique, and its integrity must be preserved for normal vision to occur. A DTH reaction in the eye, though effective in eliminating a pernicious antigen, would result in catastrophic consequences in the retina.

Consequently, a distinctive immune milieu evolved in the eye that permitted immune responsiveness to antigens, while at the same time it preserved the integrity of the retina and the visual axis. Specifically, the immune effectors that the eye uses to combat disease are cytotoxic T cells and noncomplement-fixing antibodies. DTH and complement-fixing antibodies are inhibited locally and systemically. The systemic inhibition of these immune effectors ensures that no extraocular immune response is generated against antigens that can cross-react with those in the eye; such a systemic response could become potent enough to enter the eye, overcome its immunosuppressive environment, and destroy the retina. Cytotoxic T cells and noncomplement-fixing antibodies are not as competent as DTH in removing antigens. Thus, the eye makes, as Streilein termed it, a "dangerous compromise" with the immune system to preserve retinal integrity.[128]

Adverse Effects of Anterior Chamber–Associated Immune Deviation

Herpes Simplex Virus Infection.   Although humoral and cytotoxic T cell responses generally suffice in providing the eye with protection, they are ineffectual in posterior chamber HSV-1 infection. In this case, the infected eye initially appears to clear the virus effectively through the action of cytotoxic T cells and antiviral antibodies. However, these effectors are insufficient in preventing the spread of the virus through neurons to the contralateral eye, where acute retinal infection occurs leading to necrosis.

Tumor Growth.   Ironically, the action of cytotoxic T cells and antibodies effectively limits the systemic spread of ocular tumors while being ineffec-

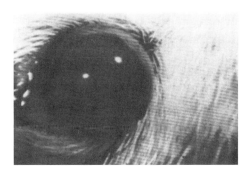

FIGURE 2.5. Anterior chamber of mouse eye filled with growing mastocytoma 10 days after intracameral injection with 10^5 cells. (Reprinted with permission from J Niederkorn, JW Streilein, JA Shadduck. Deviant immune responses to allogeneic tumors injected intracamerally and subcutaneously in mice. Invest Ophthalmol Vis Sci 1981;20:355–363. Copyright 1981, Association for Research in Vision and Ophthalmology.)

tive in eliminating the original ocular tumor, which continues to grow progressively (Figure 2.5).

Beneficial Effects of Anterior Chamber–Associated Immune Deviation

Stromal Keratitis. ACAID appears to have been an evolutionary adaptation acquired by higher vertebrates, being absent in amphibians and fish.[129] It therefore follows that its advantages should outweigh its disadvantages. In addition to the preservation of retinal integrity, other benefits of ACAID have been identified. Stromal keratitis, evident during anterior chamber HSV-1 infection, is thought to represent a DTH reaction to viral antigens in the corneal stroma as opposed to a direct toxic effect of the virus. However, this condition develops relatively infrequently (~20% of cases) in HSV infection due to the inhibition of DTH reactions in the intraocular environment.[10] Furthermore, eradication of anterior chamber HSV infection occurs despite the absence of an antiviral DTH response.

Corneal Allograft Acceptance. The high rate of acceptance of corneal allografts is thought to owe its success, in part, to ACAID. Abolishing ACAID by corneal cauterization, neovascularization, or keratoplasty was variably associated with loss of corneal, iris, and ciliary body immunosuppressive factor production, movement of Langerhans' cells into the central cornea, and leakiness of corneal neovessels.[33] Furthermore, denervation of the central cornea was also associated with the abolition of ACAID. In such animals, explants of iris and ciliary body tissues lacked the normal capacity to suppress T cell activation in vitro.[33] It is likely that disruption of neural connections to the cornea adversely affects immunosuppressive

TABLE 2.5
Clinical Significance of Anterior Chamber–Associated Immune Deviation

Adverse effects	Allows spread of herpes simplex virus type 1 (HSV-1) to contralateral eye, causing retinal necrosis
	Ineffective in eliminating ocular tumors
Beneficial effects	Prevents stromal keratitis in HSV-1 infection
	Facilitates corneal allograft acceptance
	Inhibits systemic metastases from intraocular tumors
	Prevents ocular autoimmunity

factor release by tissues lining the anterior chamber.[128] Moreover, this latter finding suggests that neurally derived factors contribute to ACAID, as mentioned earlier. This fits nicely with the demonstrated presence of neuropeptides such as VIP, CGRP, and α-MSH in aqueous humor.

Ocular Autoimmunity.   ACAID is thought to play an important role in preventing uveoretinal autoreactivity under normal and pathologic conditions and following trauma, such as in sympathetic ophthalmia. It has been shown that ACAID induction to the retinal antigens S-Ag and interphotoreceptor retinoid-binding protein (IRBP) prevented experimental autoimmune uveoretinitis in rodents.[130,131] Perhaps more clinically relevant was the finding that IRBP-induced uveoretinitis could be prevented by the in vitro ACAID-generating technique in which animals were injected with PECs previously cultured with IRBP and TGF-β. Table 2.5 summarizes the clinical significance of ACAID.

Future Directions.   The approach of using PECs to generate ACAID-inducing cells in vitro certainly holds promise for treating inflammatory eye diseases such as uveoretinitis. Because ACAID inhibits systemic, as well as ocular, DTH, it follows that this technique could conceivably be used to prevent adverse DTH-like reactions elsewhere in the body. Specifically, it is feasible that a systemic autoimmune disease that is mediated by T cells and macrophages might be preventable by such an approach. Indeed, such a strategy was used to reduce the incidence of spontaneous autoimmune type I diabetes in a rat model.[132]

References

1. Van Dooremaal JC. Die entwickelung der in grund versetzten lebenden gewebe. Albrecht von Graefes Arch Ophthalmol 1873;19:359.
2. Zahn FW. Ueber das Schicksal der in den organismus implantirten gewebe. Virchow's Arch Pathol Anat Physiol 1884;95:369–377.

3. Barker CF, Billingham RE. Immunologically privileged sites. Adv Immunol 1977;25:1–54.

4. Streilein JW, Wilbanks GA, Cousins SW. Immunoregulatory mechanisms of the eye. J Neuroimmunol 1992;39:185–200.

5. Yasunami Y, Lacy PE, Finke EH. A new site for islet transplantation—a peritoneal omental pouch. Transplantation 1983;36:181–182.

6. Riley MV. Transport of Ions and Metabolites Across the Endothelium. In DS McDevitt (ed), Cell Biology of the Eye. London. Academic Press, 1982;67.

7. Romaniuk A, Malejczyk J, Kubicka U, et al. Rejection of cartilage formed by transplanted allogeneic chondrocytes: evaluation with monoclonal antibodies. Transpl Immunol 1995;3:251–257.

8. Claas FHJ, Roelen DL, D'Amaro J, et al. The Role of HLA in Corneal Transplantation. In M Zierhut, U Pleyer, HU Thiel (eds), Immunology of Corneal Transplantation. Boston: Butterworth–Heinemann, 1994;47.

9. Reif OW, Freitag R. Studies of complexes between proteases, substrates and the protease inhibitor alpha-2-macroglobulin using capillary electrophoresis with laser-induced fluorescence detection. J Chromatogr 1995;716:363–369.

10. Streilein JW. Regional Immunology of the Eye. In JS Pepose, G Holland, K Wilhelmus (eds), Ocular Infection and Immunity. Boston: Mosby, 1995;19–32.

11. Vinores SA. Assessment of blood-retinal barrier integrity. Histol Histopathol 1995;10:141–154.

12. Prendergast RA, Iliff CE, Coskuncan NM, et al. T cell traffic and the inflammatory response in experimental autoimmune uveoretinitis. Invest Ophthalmol Vis Sci 1998;39:754–762.

13. Sainte-Marie G, Sin YM. The lymph node: structure and possible function during the immune response. Rev Can Biol 1968;27:191–207.

14. De Arruda MS, Montenegro MR. The hamster cheek pouch: an immunologically privileged site suitable to the study of granulomatous infection. Rev Inst Med Trop Sao Paulo 1995;37:303–309.

15. Hamasaki M, Kumabe T. Three-dimensional structure of two different lymphatic spaces in rat testis, and the route of flow fluxes of their lymphatic fluids. Acta Anat Nippon 1994;69:669–683.

16. McCullough DL. Experimental lymphangiography. Experience with direct medium injection into the parenchyma of the rat testis and prostate. Invest Urol 1975;13:211–219.

17. Johanson CE. Ventricles and Cerebrospinal Fluid. In PM Conn (ed), Neuroscience in Medicine. Philadelphia: Lippincott–Raven, 1995;190.

18. Bill A. The role of ciliary blood flow and ultrafiltration in aqueous humor formation. Exp Eye Res 1973;16:287–298.

19. Yelavarthi KK, Schmidt CM, Ehlenfeldt RG, et al. Cellular distribution of HLA-G mRNA in transgenic mouse placentas. J Immunol 1993;151: 3638–3645.

20. Ulbrecht M, Rehberger B, Strobel I, et al. HLA-G: expression in human keratinocytes in vitro and in human skin in vivo. Eur J Immunol 1994;24: 176–180.

21. Athanassakis I, Aifantis Y, Makrygiannakis A, et al. Placental tissue from human miscarriages expresses class II HLA-DR antigens. Am J Reprod Immunol 1995;34:281–287.

22. Neumann H, Cavalie A, Jenne DE, Wekerle H. Induction of MHC class I genes in neurons. Science 1995;269:549–552.

23. Fabry Z, Raine CS, Hart MN. Nervous tissue as an immune compartment: the dialect of the immune response in the CNS. Immunol Today 1994;15: 218–224.

24. Pollanen P, Jahnukainen K, Punnonen J, Sainio-Pollanen S. Ontogeny of immunosuppressive activity, MHC antigens and leukocytes in the rat testis. J Reprod Immunol 1992;21:257–274.

25. Lynch MG, Peeler JS, Brown RH, Niederkorn JY. Expression of HLA class I and II antigens on cells of the human trabecular meshwork. Ophthalmology 1987;94:851–857.

26. Tripathi BJ, Tripathi RC, Wong P, Raja S. Expression of HLA by the human trabecular meshwork and corneal endothelium. Exp Eye Res 1990;51:269–276.

27. Bakker M, Grumet FC, Feltkamp TEW, Kijlstra A. HLA-antigens in the human uvea. Doc Ophthalmol 1986;61:271–279.

28. Benson MT, Shepherd L, Cottam D, et al. The expression of class I major histocompatibility antigens by human retinal pigment epithelium in vitro. Graefe's Arch Clin Exp Ophthalmol 1992;230:184–187.

29. Martin WD, Egan RM, Stevens JL, Woodward JG. Lens-specific expression of a major histocompatibility complex class I molecule disrupts normal lens development and induces cataracts in transgenic mice. Invest Ophthalmol Vis Sci 1995;36:1144–1154.

30. Streilein JW, Toews GB, Bergstresser PR. Corneal allografts fail to express Ia antigens. Nature 1979;282:326–327.

31. Niederkorn JY, Peeler JS, Mellon J. Phagocytosis of particulate antigens by corneal epithelial cells stimulates interleukin-I secretion and migration of Langerhans' cells into the central cornea. Reg Immunol 1989;2:83–90.

32. Roussel TJ, Osato MS, Wilhemus KR. Corneal Langerhans' cells migration following ocular contact sensitivity. Cornea 1983;2:27–30.

33. Streilein JW, Bradley D, Sano Y, Sonoda Y. Immunosuppressive properties of tissues obtained from eyes with experimentally manipulated corneas. Invest Ophthalmol Vis Sci 1996;37:413–424.

34. Williamson JSP, DiMarco S, Streilein JW. Immunobiology of Langerhans' cells on the ocular surface. I. Langerhans' cells within the central cornea interfere with induction of anterior chamber associated immune deviation. Invest Ophthalmol Vis Sci 1987;28:1527–1532.

35. Williamson JSP, Bradley D, Streilein JW. Immunoregulatory properties of bone marrow-derived cells in the iris and ciliary body. Immunology 1989;67: 96–102.

36. Knisely TL, Anderson TM, Sherwood ME, et al. Morphologic and ultrastructural examination of I-A+ cells in the murine iris. Invest Ophthalmol Vis Sci 1991;32:2423–2431.

37. McMenamin PG, Holthouse I, Holt PG. Class II major histocompatibility complex (Ia) antigen-bearing dendritic cells within the iris and ciliary body of the rat eye: distribution, phenotype and relation to retinal microglia. Immunology 1992;77:385–393.

38. McMenamin PG, Crewe J, Morrison S, Holt PG. Immunomorphologic studies of macrophages and MHC class II positive dendritic cells in the iris and ciliary body of the rat, mouse, and human eye. Invest Ophthalmol Vis Sci 1994;35:3234–3250.

39. Flugel C, Kinne RW, Streilein JW, Lutjen-Drecoll E. Distinctive distribution of bone marrow derived cells in the anterior segment of human eyes. Curr Eye Res 1992;11:1173–1184.

40. Penfold PL, Provis JM, Liew SC. Human retinal microglia express phenotypic characteristics in common with dendritic antigen-presenting cells. J Neuroimmunol 1993;45:183–191.

41. Caspi RR, Roberge FG, Nussenblatt RB. Organ-resident, non-lymphoid cells suppress proliferation of autoimmune T-helper lymphocytes. Science 1987;237:1029–1032.

42. Streilein JW, Bradley D. Analysis of immunosuppressive properties of iris and ciliary body cells and their secretory products. Invest Ophthalmol Vis Sci 1991;32:2700–2710.

43. Benezra D, Sachs U. Growth factors in aqueous humor or normal and inflamed eyes of rabbits. Invest Ophthalmol Vis Sci 1973;13:868–870.

44. Kaiser CJ, Ksander BR, Streilein JW. Inhibition of lymphocyte proliferation by aqueous humor. Reg Immunol 1989;2:42–49.

45. Streilen JW. Ocular immune privilege in the immunosuppressive intraocular microenvironment. Ocul Immunol Inflamm 1995;3:139–143.

46. Ottaway CA. Vasoactive intestinal peptide as a modulator of lymphocyte and immune function. Ann N Y Acad Sci 1988;527:486–500.

47. Ganea D, Sun L. Vasoactive intestinal peptide downregulates the expression of IL-2 but not of INF-γ from stimulated murine T lymphocytes. J Neuroimmunol 1993;47:147–158.

48. Ishioka C, Yoshida A, Kimata H, Mikawa H. Vasoactive intestinal peptide stimulates immunoglobulin production and growth of human B cells. Clin Exp Immunol 1992;878:504–508.

49. Grimes PA, Uddoh C, Koeberlein B, Stone RA. Helospectin-like immunoreactivity in the rat eye and pterygopalatine ganglion. Neurosci Lett 1995;183:108–111.

50. Taylor AW, Streilein JW, Cousins SW. Identification of α-melanocyte stimulating hormone as a potential immunosuppressive factor in aqueous humor. Curr Eye Res 1992;11:1199–1206.

51. Lipton JM. Modulation of host defense by the neuropeptide α-MSH. Yale J Biol Med 1990;63:173–182.

52. Asahina A, Hosoi J, Beissert S, et al. Inhibition of delayed type and contact hypersensitivity by calcitonin gene-related peptide. J Immunol 1995;154:3056–3061.

53. Wahlestedt C, Beding B, Ekman R, et al. Calcitonin gene-related peptide in the eye: release by sensory nerve stimulation and effects associated with neurogenic inflammation. Regul Pept 1986;16:107–115.

54. Knisely TL, Hosoi J, Nazareno R, Granstein RD. The presence of biologically significant concentrations of glucocorticoids but little or no cortisol binding globulin within aqueous humor: relevance to immune privilege in the anterior chamber of the eye. Invest Ophthalmol Vis Sci 1994;35:3711–3723.

55. Apte RS, Niederkorn JY. Isolation and characterization of a unique natural killer cell inhibitory factor present in the anterior chamber of the eye. J Immunol 1996;156:2667–2673.

56. Roberts AB, Anzano MA, Lamb LC, et al. New class of transforming growth factors potentiated by epidermal growth factor: isolation from non-neoplastic tissues. Proc Natl Acad Sci U S A 1981;78:5339–5343.

57. Barnard JA, Lyons RM, Moses HM. The cell biology of transforming growth factor-β. Biochim Biophys Acta 1990;1032:79–87.

58. Lawrence DA. Transforming growth factor-β: an overview. Kidney Int Suppl 1995;49:S19–523.

59. Bombara C, Ignotz RA. TGF-Beta inhibits proliferation of and promotes differentiation of human promonocytic leukemia cells. J Cell Physiol 1992;153:30–37.

60. Massague J. The transforming growth factor-β family. Annu Rev Cell Biol 1990;6:597–641.

61. Sporn MB, Roberts AB. Transforming growth factor-beta. Multiple actions and potential clinical applications. JAMA 1989;262:938–941.

62. Shalaby MR, Ammann AJ. Suppression of immune cell function in vitro by recombinant human transforming growth factor-beta. Cell Immunol 1988;112:343–350.

63. Ellingsworth LR, Nakayama D, Segarini P, et al. Transforming growth factor-betas are equipotent growth inhibitors of interleukin-1 induced thymocyte proliferation. Cell Immunol 1988;114:41–54.

64. Kehrl JH, Wakefield LM, Roberts AB, et al. Production of transforming growth factor beta by human T lymphocytes and its potential role in the regulation of T cell function. J Exp Med 1986;163:1037–1050.

65. Kehrl JH, Roberts AB, Wakefield LM, et al. Transforming growth factor beta is an important immunomodulatory protein for human B lymphocytes. J Immunol 1986;137:3855–3860.

66. Ranges GE, Figari IS, Espevik T, Palladino MA. Inhibition of cytotoxic T cell development by transforming growth factor beta and reversal by recombinant tumor necrosis factor alpha. J Exp Med 1987;166:991–998.

67. Fontana A, Frei K, Bodmer S, et al. Transforming growth factor-beta inhibits the generation of cytotoxic T cells in virus-infected mice. J Immunol 1989;143:3230–3234.

68. Rook AH, Kehrl JH, Wakefield LM, et al. Effects of transforming growth factor beta on the functions of natural killer cells: depressed cytolytic activity and blunting of interferon responsiveness. J Immunol 1986;136:3916–3920.

69. Zuber P, Kuppner MC, De Tribolet N. Transforming growth factor-β2 down-regulates HLA-DR antigen expression on human malignant glioma cells. Eur J Immunol 1988;18:1623–1626.

70. Gupta A, Monroy D, Ji Z, et al. Transforming growth factor beta-1 and beta-2 in human tear fluid. Curr Eye Res 1996;15:605–614.

71. Pircher R, Jullien P, Lawrence DA. β-Transforming growth factor is stored in human blood platelets as a latent high molecular weight complex. Biochem Biophys Res Commun 1986;136:30–37.

72. Odekon LE, Blasi F, Rifkin DB. Requirement for receptor-bound urokinase in plasmin-dependent cellular conversion of latent TGF-beta to TGF-beta. J Cell Physiol 1994;158:398–407.

73. Sato Y, Rifkin DB. Inhibition of endothelial cell movement by pericytes and smooth muscle cells: activation of latent transforming growth factor-β1-like molecule by plasmin during co-culture. J Cell Biol 1989;109:309–315.

74. Miyazono K, Ichijo H, Heldin C-H. Transforming growth factor-β: latent forms, binding proteins and receptors. Growth Factors 1993;8:11–22.

75. Jampel HD, Roche N, Stark WJ, Roberts AB. Transforming growth factor-β in human aqueous humor. Curr Eye Res 1990;9:963–969.

76. Granstein RD, Staszewski R, Knisely TL, et al. Aqueous humor contains transforming growth factor-beta and a small (<3500 daltons) inhibitor of thymocyte proliferation. J Immunol 1990;144:3021–3027.

77. Cousins SW, McCabe MM, Danielpour D, Streilein JW. Identification of transforming growth factor-beta as an immunosuppressive factor in aqueous humor. Invest Ophthalmol Vis Sci 1991;32:2201–2211.

78. Helbig H, Gurley RC, Palestine AG, et al. Dual effect of ciliary body cells on T lymphocyte proliferation. Eur J Immunol 1990;20:2457–2463.

79. Knisely TL, Bleicher PA, Vibbard CA, Granstein RD. Production of latent transforming growth factor-beta and other inhibitory factors by cultured murine iris and ciliary body cells. Curr Eye Res 1991;10:761–771.

80. de Boer JH, Limpens J, Orengo-Nania S, et al. A. Low mature TGF-beta 2 levels in aqueous humor during uveitis. Invest Ophthalmol Vis Sci 1994;35:3702–3710.

81. Tanihara H, Yoshida M, Matsumoto M, Yoshimura N. Identification of transforming growth factor-β expressed in cultured human retinal pigment epithelial cells. Invest Ophthalmol Vis Sci 1993;34:413–419.

82. Pasquale LR, Dorman-Pease ME, Lutty GA, et al. Immunolocalization of TGF-β1, TGF-β2, and TGF-β3 in the anterior segment of the human eye. Invest Ophthalmol Vis Sci 1993;34:23–30.

83. Anderson DH, Guerin CJ, Hageman GS, et al. Distribution of transforming growth factor-beta isoforms in the mammalian retina. J Neurosci Res 1995;42:63–79.

84. Smalley DM, Fitzgerald JE, Taylor DM, et al. Tissue plasminogen activator activity in human aqueous humor. Invest Ophthalmol Vis Sci 1994;35:48–53.

85. Wang Y, Taylor DM, Smalley DM, et al. Increased basal levels of free plasminogen activator activity found in human aqueous humor. Invest Ophthalmol Vis Sci 1994;35:3561–3566.

86. Wang Y, Gillies C, Cone RE, O'Rourke J. Extravascular secretion of t-PA by the intact superfused choroid. Invest Ophthalmol Vis Sci 1995;36:1625–1632.

87. Park SS, Li L, Korn TS, et al. Effect of transforming growth factor-beta on plasminogen activator production of cultured human uveal melanoma cells. Curr Eye Res 1996;15:755–763.

88. Griffith TS, Brunner T, Fletcher SM, et al. Fas ligand-induced apoptosis as a mechanism of immune privilege. Science 1995;270:1189–1192.

89. Wilson SE, Li Q, Weng J, et al. The fas-fas ligand system and other modulators of apoptosis in the cornea. Invest Ophthalmol Vis Sci 1996;37: 1582–1592.

90. Bhandoola A, Yui K, Siegel RM, et al. Gld and Lpr mice: single gene mutant models for failed self tolerance. Int Rev Immunol 1994;11:231–244.

91. Bellgrau D, Gold D, Selawry H, et al. A role for CD95 ligand in preventing graft rejection. Nature 1995;377:630–632.

92. Kaplan HJ, Streilein JW. Immune response to immunization via the anterior chamber of the eye. I. F1 lymphocyte-induced immune deviation. J Immunol 1977;118:809–814.

93. Wilbanks GA, Mammolenti M, Streilein JW. Studies on the induction of ACAID. II. Eye-derived cells participate in generating blood-borne signals that induce ACAID. J Immunol 1991;146:3018–3024.

94. Wilbanks GA, Streilein JW. Characterization of suppressor cells in ACAID induced by soluble antigen. Evidence of two functionally and phenotypically distinct T-suppressor cell populations. Immunology 1990;71:383–389.

95. Hara Y, Caspi RR, Wiggert B, et al. Suppression of experimental autoimmune uveitis in mice by induction of ACAID with interphotoreceptor retinoid-binding protein. J Immunol 1992;148:1685–1692.

96. Waldrep JC, Kaplan HJ. Anterior chamber-associated immune deviation induced by TNP-splenocytes (TNP-ACAID). II. Suppressor T-cell networks. Invest Ophthalmol Vis Sci 1983;24:1339–1345.

97. Atherton SS, Kanter MY, Streilein JW. ACAID requires early replication of HSV-1 in the injected eye. Curr Eye Res 1991;10(suppl):75–80.

98. Niederkorn JY, Mayhew E. Role of splenic B cells in the immune privilege of the anterior chamber of the eye. Eur J Immunol 1995;25:2783–2787.

99. Bando Y, Ksander BR, Streilein JW. Characterization of specific T helper cell activity in mice bearing alloantigenic tumors in the anterior chamber of the eye. Eur J Immunol 1991;21:1923–1931.

100. Niederkorn J, Streilein JW, Shadduck JA. Deviant immune responses to allogenic tumors injected intracamerally and subcutaneously in mice. Invest Ophthalmol Vis Sci 1980;20:355–363.

101. Streilein JW, Niederkorn JY, Shadduck JA. Systemic immune unresponsiveness induced in adult mice by anterior chamber presentation of minor histocompatibility antigens. J Exp Med 1980;152:1121–1125.

102. Niederkorn JY, Streilein JW. Alloantigens placed into the anterior chamber of the eye induce specific suppression of delayed type hypersensitivity but normal cytotoxic T lymphocyte responses. J Immunol 1983;131:2670–2674.

103. Streilein JW, Niederkorn JY. Characterization of the suppressor cells responsible for ACAID induced in BALB/c mice by P815 cells. J Immunol 1984;20:603–622.

104. Wilbanks GA, Streilein JW. Distinctive humoral responses following anterior chamber and intravenous administration of soluble antigen: evidence for active suppression of IgG2a-secreting B cells. Immunology 1990;71:566–572.

105. Asherson GL, Stone SH. Selective and specific inhibition of 24 hour skin reactions in the guinea-pig. I. Immune deviation: description of the phenomenon and the effect of splenectomy. Immunology 1965;9:205–217.

106. Wilbanks GA, Streilein JW. Studies on the induction of ACAID. I. Evidence that an antigen-specific, ACAID-inducing, cell associated signal exists in the peripheral blood. J Immunol 1991;146:2610–2617.

107. Streilein JW, Niederkorn JY. Induction of ACAID requires an intact, functional spleen. J Exp Med 1981;153:1058–1067.

108. Ferguson TA, Hayashi JD, Kaplan HJ. The immune response and the eye. III. Anterior chamber-associated immune deviation can be adoptively transferred by serum. J Immunol 1989;143:821–826.

109. Hara Y, Okamoto S, Rouse B, Streilein JW. Evidence that peritoneal exudate cells cultured with eye-derived fluids are the proximate antigen-presenting cells in immune deviation of the ocular type. J Immunol 1993;151:5162–5171.

110. Wilbanks GA, Streilein JW. Fluid from immune privileged sites endow macrophages with the capacity to induce antigen-specific immune deviation via a mechanism involving TGF-β. Eur J Immunol 1992;22:1031–1036.

111. Wilbanks GA, Mammolenti MM, Streilein JW. Studies on the induction of ACAID. III. Induction of anterior chamber-associated immune deviation depends upon intraocular transforming growth factor beta. Eur J Immunol 1992;22:165–174.

112. Okano Y, Hara Y, Yao Y-F, Tano Y. In Vitro-ACAID Induction by Culturing Blood Monocytes with Transforming Growth Factor-Beta. In RB Nussenblatt, RR Whitcup, RR Caspi, I Gery (eds), Advances in Ocular Immunology. Bethesda, MD: Elsevier Science BV, 1994;199–202.

113. Takeuchi M, Kosiewicz MM, Alard P, Streilein JW. On the mechanisms by which transforming growth factor-beta 2 alters antigen-presenting abilities of macrophages on T cell activation. Eur J Immunol 1997;27:1648–1656.

114. Takeuchi M, Alard P, Streilein JW. TGF-beta promotes immune deviation by altering accessory signals of antigen-presenting cells. J Immunol 1998;160:1589–1597.

115. Streilein JW. Molecular basis of ACAID. Ocul Immunol Inflamm 1997;5:217–218.

116. Streilein JW. Regulation of ocular immune responses. Eye 1997;11:171–175.

117. Griffith TS, Herndon JM, Lima J, et al. The immune response and the eye. TCR α-chain related molecules regulate the systemic immunity to antigen presented in the eye. Int Immunol 1995;7:1617–1625.

118. Niederkorn JY. Exogenous recombinant interleukin-2 abrogates anterior chamber-associated immune deviation. Transplantation 1987;43:523–528.

119. Benson JL, Niederkorn JY. Interleukin-1 abrogates anterior chamber-associated immune deviation. Invest Ophthalmol Vis Sci 1990;31:2123–2128.
120. Ferguson TA, Herndon JM, Dube P. The immune response and the eye. IV. A role for tumor necrosis factor alpha in anterior chamber associated immune deviation. Invest Ophthalmol Vis Sci 1994;35:2643–2651.
121. D'Orazio TJ, Niederkorn JY. A novel role for TGF-β and IL-10 in the induction of immune privilege. J Immunol 1998;160:2089–2098.
122. Geiger K, Sarvetnick N. Local production of IFN-γ abrogates the intraocular immune privilege in transgenic mice and prevents the induction of ACAID. J Immunol 1994;153:5239–5246.
123. Cousins SW, Trattler WB, Streilein JW. Immune privilege and suppression of immunogenic inflammation in the anterior chamber of the eye. Curr Eye Res 1991;10:287–297.
124. Kripke ML. Immunological unresponsiveness induced by ultraviolet light. Immunol Rev 1984;80:87–102.
125. Ferguson TA, Hayashi JD, Kaplan HJ. Regulation of the systemic immune response by visible light and the eye. FASEB J 1988;2:3017–3021.
126. Ferguson TA, Fletcher S, Herndon J, Griffith TS. Neuropeptides modulate immune deviation induced via the anterior chamber of the eye. J Immunol 1995;155:1746–1756.
127. Eichhorn M, Horneber M, Streilein JW, Lutjen-Drecoll E. Anterior associated immune deviation elicited via primate eyes. Invest Ophthalmol Vis Sci 1993;34:2926–2930.
128. Streilein JW. Immune regulation and the eye: a dangerous compromise. FASEB J 1987;1:199–208.
129. Sano Y, Streilein JW. Effects of Corneal Surgical Wounds on Ocular Immune Privilege. In RB Nussenblatt, SM Whitcup, RR Caspi, I Gery (eds), Advances in Ocular Immunology. Bethesda, MD: Elsevier Science BV, 1994;207–210.
130. Hara Y, Caspi RR, Wiggert B, et al. Suppression of experimental autoimmune uveitis in mice by induction of anterior chamber associated immune deviation with interphotoreceptor retinoid binding protein. J Immunol 1992;148:1685–1692.
131. Mizuno K, Clark AF, Streilein JW. Ocular injection of retinal S antigen: suppression of autoimmune uveitis. Invest Ophthalmol Vis Sci 1989;30:772–774.
132. Koevary SB. Prevention of diabetes in BB/Wor rats by injection of peritoneal exudate cells cultured in the presence of transforming growth factor beta (TGF-β) and islet cells. Diabetes Res 1994;27:1–14.

CHAPTER 3

Immunity of Specific Ocular Tissues

If you have tears, prepare to shed them now.
—William Shakespeare, *Julius Caesar*

For an infectious agent to enter the body, an epithelial barrier must be breached. These barriers exist in the skin, mucous membranes, gastrointestinal tract, respiratory tract, and on the anterior surface of the eye. In each of these regions, the anti-infectious nature of the epithelium is bolstered by the presence of various cytokines, antibodies, and other proteins.

When a microorganism gains a foothold in subepithelial tissues, it can divide and establish a locus of infection that can ultimately be disseminated throughout the body. In the case of the eye, certain intraocular tissues such as the uveal tract can succumb to infections that enter the body through regions other than the eye and that are brought to the eye by the vasculature. In this chapter, the specific mechanisms by which infectious agents are prevented from directly penetrating into the ocular tissues through the anterior surface of the eye are discussed, followed by an analysis of the immune response to infection of the cornea, conjunctiva, sclera, choroid, ciliary body, iris, and retina.

Role of Tear Film in Preventing Ocular Infection

The tear film performs several important functions, listed in Table 3.1, including lubrication of the anterior surface of the eye, maintenance of a smooth optical surface by adherence to the corneal surface, removal of cellular and particulate debris, low-level nourishment of the corneal and conjunctival epithelial cells, and elimination of pathogenic organisms.[1]

TABLE 3.1
Functions of the Tear Film

Moistens and lubricates the eye
Contributes to the establishment of a smooth optical surface
Maintains integrity of corneal and conjunctival epithelia
Removes desquamated corneal cells and bacteria
Prevents microbial colonization on the ocular surface
Provides nominal nourishment to corneal epithelium

Source: Modified with permission from R Stein, JJ Hurwitz. Anatomy and Physiology of Tear Secretion. In JJ Hurwitz (ed), The Lacrimal System. Philadelphia: Lippincott–Raven, 1966;1.

The osmolarity and pH (7.4) of tears are nearly identical to that of plasma.[2] The lacrimal, accessory lacrimal, and sebaceous glands, as well as conjunctival goblet and epithelial cells, all contribute to the secretion of tears. The lacrimal and accessory lacrimal glands can each constitutively produce tears at a slow, basal rate, and can also rapidly secrete larger volumes of stored tear fluid reflexively in response to neurologic input.[3] Over the course of 16 wakeful hours, it has been estimated that between 0.50 and 1.25 ml of tear fluid are produced.[4] A schematic representation of the sources of the entire tear film is shown in Figure 3.1.

The tear film is composed of three distinct layers, each of which contributes either directly or indirectly to the film's role in maintaining a sterile environment on the surface of the eye.

Innermost, Mucous Layer

The innermost, or mucous, layer is produced by conjunctival goblet and epithelial cells[5] and closely adheres to the surface of the globe. The corneal apical cells exhibit a glycocalyx that attaches loosely to this layer and also binds to immunoglobulins in the aqueous layer.[6] Glycoproteins in the mucous layer facilitate the spreading of the aqueous tear film over the eye.

What role does the mucous layer play in ocular immunity? It is the site of binding of immunoglobulins (produced in the aqueous layer) to the corneal cells. It also plays an indirect role, hydrating the corneal and conjunctival epithelia and coating them with a protective layer of mucus. There have been reports that certain mucins have antiviral effects; specifically, intestinal mucins were shown to be potent inhibitors of rotavirus replication.[7] Thus, a role for tear film mucins in the prevention of viral replication on the surface of the eye may yet be described. Although a deficiency in tear mucus was thought to play a role in cicatricial pemphigoid and Stevens-Johnson syndrome, several studies have shown that, in fact, substantial amounts of ocular mucous glycoprotein are present in the eyes of these patients.[8,9]

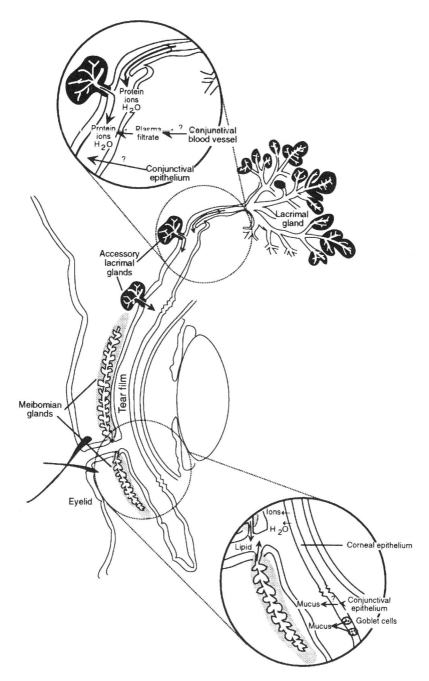

FIGURE 3.1.   Schematic of the orbital glands and ocular epithelia that secrete the different layers of the tear film. (Reprinted with slight modification, with permission, from DA Dartt. Physiology of Tear Production. In MA Lemp, R Marguardt [eds], The Dry Eye: A Comprehensive Guide. New York: Springer-Verlag, 1992;2.)

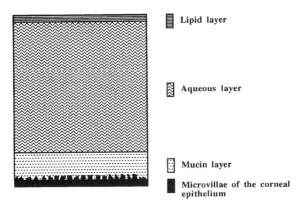

FIGURE 3.2.   Schematic representation of the tear film. (Reprinted with permission from R Stein, JJ Hurwitz. Anatomy and Physiology of Tear Secretion. In JJ Hurwitz [ed], The Lacrimal System. Philadelphia: Lippincott–Raven, 1996;2.)

Middle, Aqueous Layer

The middle layer, also called the *aqueous layer*, is the thickest; it accounts for about 90% of the entire tear film (Figure 3.2).[10] It is 8 µm thick and contains approximately 8 µl of fluid. The aqueous layer contains numerous proteins that have antimicrobial properties.

Lactoferrin

Lactoferrin, produced by the acinar cells of the lacrimal gland, binds iron, which is required for bacterial growth, and thus has bacteriostatic and bactericidal properties. Other actions of lactoferrin include prevention of cellular free radical damage,[11] inhibition of complement C3 convertase[12] and complement-mediated red blood cell lysis, and intensification of the effects of antibody.[13]

It is becoming clear that many microorganisms can counteract the effects of lactoferrin by secreting iron chelators (called *siderophores*) that compete with lactoferrin for iron.[11] Derivatives of lactoferrin, called *lactoferricins*, have been shown to have antimicrobial activity independent of iron chelation.[14] Whether such compounds play a role in the antimicrobial action of tears is unknown.

Lysozyme

The enzyme lysozyme is produced by type A cells in the lacrimal gland. It is a hydrolase that makes up nearly one-fourth of the total protein in tears[15] and that works best in near-neutral pH. It has the ability to lyse the cell wall of certain gram-positive organisms by cleaving the bond between

TABLE 3.2
Antimicrobial Functions of Secretory IgA

Agglutination
Prevention of microbial attachment
Inactivation of bacterial enzymes or toxins
Antibody-dependent cell-mediated cytotoxicity
Opsonization

---

muramic acid and glucosamine residues. Unfortunately, one of the most common ocular gram-positive bacteria, *Staphylococcus aureus*, is not susceptible to lysis by lysozyme.[16] Lysozyme has also been shown to bolster the activity of immunoglobulin A (IgA) antibody against gram-negative bacteria.[17]

Immunoglobulin A

IgA plays an important role in ocular surface immunity. Of the five antibody isotypes, IgA is produced in the greatest abundance, though relatively little of it is present in serum. Instead, it is secreted through epithelial cells in the gastrointestinal tract, bronchial mucosa, lactating breast, parotid gland, and lacrimal gland to enter the gastrointestinal lumen, bronchial lumen, milk, saliva, and tears, respectively. Because it is secreted into body fluids and cavities rather than into the blood, this immunoglobulin is referred to as *secretory IgA* and in that form consists of two IgA molecules coupled to a polypeptide chain called the *J chain* and to a protein called *secretory piece*. In mother's milk, it confers passive immunity to the neonate. In all other secretions, it binds to bacteria and viruses and prevents them from adhering to mucosal surfaces by direct interference with their binding sites or by agglutination. Specifically in the eye, this facilitates the washing away of microorganisms by the tear fluid. IgA also prevents infection by inactivation of bacterial enzymes and toxins, by opsonization, and possibly by antibody-dependent cell-mediated cytotoxicity (ADCC) (Table 3.2). IgA cannot bind to complement proteins and thus does not have the capacity to activate complement by the classical cascade.[17]

Plasma cells located beneath secretory cells lining the acini in the lacrimal gland are the source of IgA destined for inclusion in tear fluid. The two cytokines thought to play a role in the isotype switch to IgA in these cells are transforming growth factor–beta (TGF-β) and interleukin-5 (IL-5). These cells secrete dimeric IgA, which is held together by the polypeptide J chain. This complex then binds, by way of its J chain and the heavy chains of each of its IgA monomeric units, to the protein secretory component, which is synthesized by lacrimal gland acinar cells and is expressed on their basal and lateral surface. One-sixth of this protein is associated with the membrane of the acinar cell, whereas the rest of the molecule exists as an extracellular domain. After binding of dimeric IgA to secretory component, the complex is endocytosed and then transcytosed in vesicles to the acinar lumen where the extracellular domain of secretory component, carrying the IgA molecule, is proteolytically cleaved and released, leaving behind the membrane-associated component (Figure 3.3). The portion of secretory component that remains attached to the IgA dimer is referred to as *secretory piece* and plays a role in protecting the IgA dimer from degradation by bacterial proteases. This protection is generally incomplete, especially when the complex is attacked by proteases elaborated by *Streptococcus* and *Neisseria* bacteria. It should be noted that although the above mechanism for immunoglobulin transport across the lacrimal gland epithelium primarily shuttles IgA into the lumen, it can also be used to transport pentameric IgM in small amounts.

It is curious that topical ocular immunization results in a reduction in tear IgA levels. Yet, administration of antigen by the gastrointestinal route raises specific IgA levels in tears.[18] The suggested sequence of events that leads to the production of antigen-specific IgA in tears is initial trapping of antigen on the surface of the eye, its drainage into the nose and gastrointestinal tract, stimulation of immune B cells in Peyer's patches in the distal ileum, the homing of these cells to the lacrimal gland by way of the mesenteric lymph nodes and thoracic duct, and, finally, the differentiation of these B cells into IgA-secreting plasma cells (Figure 3.4). In many other tissues, lymphocytes home to their targets by binding to endothelial adhesion molecules, called *vascular addressins*, on high endothelial venules (HEVs) in the target region. However, this does not appear to be the case in the lacrimal gland. Instead, the data suggest a direct interaction of lymphocytes with molecules on the acinar epithelial cells.[19]

It should be noted that although IgA is the predominant antibody isotype in tears, in cases of ocular inflammation, it is often joined by IgG, which leaks with other serum proteins from the vasculature in the inflamed eye.

Miscellaneous Proteins in the Aqueous Layer

Beta-lysin is a bactericidal cationic protein of thrombocytic origin that is found in tears and aqueous humor.[20] The mechanism of its bactericidal activity appears to be the inhibition of bacterial catalase and peroxidase[21] and disruption of the bacterial cell membrane. Complement proteins are also present in tears. Specifically, in the closed eye, proteins C1q, C3, factor B, C4, C5, and C9 are detected, whereas only C3, factor B, and C4 are detected in the open eye and reflex tears.[22] Anticomplement proteins are also present. Lactoferrin, present in all tear types, inhibits C3 convertase, and decay-accelerating factor (DAF) found in closed eye tears accelerates the dissociation of classical and alternative pathway C3 convertases.[22] Many other enzymatic

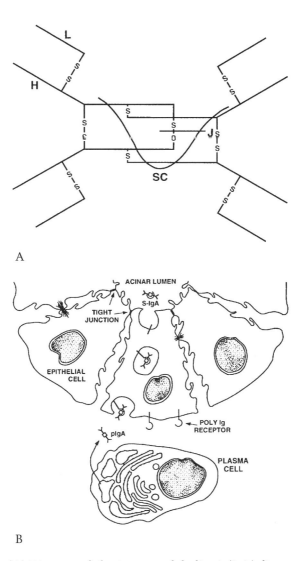

A

B

FIGURE 3.3.   (A) Diagram of the immunoglobulin A (IgA) dimer and its associated J chain (J) and secretory component (SC). (L = light chains; H = heavy chains; S
= intrachain and intercahin disulfide bonds.) (B) Pathway for IgA production and
secretion in the lacrimal gland (poly IgA is IgA dimer). (Reprinted with permission
from RM Franklin, PC Montgomery. Lacrimal Gland Immunology. In JS Pepose,
GN Holland, KR Wilhelmus [eds], Ocular Infection and Immunity. St. Louis:
Mosby–Year Book, 1992;134.)

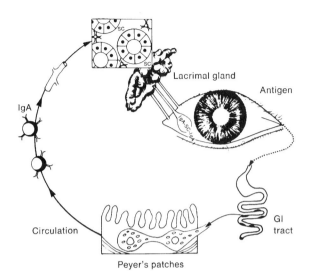

FIGURE 3.4.   Role of gastrointestinal (GI) mucosal immune system in immunoglobulin A (IgA) production in the lacrimal gland. (SC = secretory component.) (Reprinted
in modified form with permission from MR Allansmith. The Eye and Immunology.
St. Louis: Mosby, 1982;108.)

proteins are present in tears, including some that are lacking in certain
inborn errors of metabolism such as Tay-Sachs disease.[23]

Aqueous Constituents in Closed versus Open Eyes

It is important to note that the constituents in the aqueous tear film vary
depending on whether the eye has been in a sustained open or closed posi-
tion. The open eye aqueous tear fluid is rich in lysozyme, lactoferrin, and a
tear-specific prealbumin called *lipocalin*, with only low levels of IgA.[24,25]
With the restriction in tear flow that is associated with eye closure, the tear
fluid constituency changes to one containing elevated levels of both IgA[3]
and exudated serum proteins. Complement proteins are activated and neutrophils are recruited into the area, resulting in a subclinical state of inflammation.[26] This set of circumstances helps to prevent microbial adhesion
and infection. Ocular damage due to the action of complement is prevented,
by the action of DAF released in closed eye tear fluid as well as by vit-
ronectin, an adhesive glycoprotein, exudated from serum.[27] Damage caused
by mediators released from recruited neutrophils is prevented by the release
of protease inhibitors such as alpha$_1$-antitrypsin.[3]

Outer Lipid Layer

The outer lipid layer is the thinnest of the three tear film layers, measuring
only 0.1 μm. It consists of a variety of lipid constituents, including waxy

esters, triglycerides, and free fatty acids secreted by the meibomian glands and the accessory sebaceous glands of Zeis and Moll. By decreasing the evaporation of the underlying aqueous layer, the lipid layer contributes indirectly to the antimicrobial nature of the tear fluid.

Corneal Immunology

The cornea is one of the ocular immune privileged sites (see Chapter 2). Contributing to its privilege is the absence of a vascular supply and lymphatic drainage and the lack of antigen-presenting cells in the central cornea. Furthermore, the cornea has been shown to produce immunosuppressive factors.[28] One could thus assume that immunologic reactions do not occur in the cornea, but this is not the case. The clinical conditions of epithelial and stromal keratitis, subepithelial opacities, and keratic precipitates point to an immunologically reactive cornea.

Corneal tissues have the capacity to secrete a multitude of cytokines and other immune activating factors such as IL-1, IL-6, IL-8, tumor necrosis factor–alpha (TNF-α), interferon-gamma (IFN-γ), complement protein C5a, and prostaglandins.[29–32] Various conditions have been shown to result in the release of these cytokines. For example, phagocytosis of certain antigens by corneal epithelial cells stimulates their release of IL-1 and results in the migration into the central cornea of Langerhans' cells from the limbus.[33] Similarly, infection of human corneal stromal fibroblasts with herpes simplex virus (HSV) leads to the synthesis of IL-8, which may account for neutrophil infiltration in herpetic keratitis.[34] Langerhans' cells can also migrate into the central cornea in response to chemical irritants[35] or localized damage.[36] Corneal endothelial cells constitutively express the adhesion molecules intercellular adhesion molecule–1 (ICAM-1) and CD44, which play a role in lymphocyte binding to, and entrapment by, HEVs.[37,38] Finally, corneal epithelial cells were shown to express class II histocompatibility antigens and stimulate an immune response after IFN-γ treatment.[39]

Immunoglobulins also play a role in corneal immunity. IgM, IgG, and IgA are all found in the cornea. In the immunologically privileged central cornea, the IgG isotype predominates, diffusing there from fenestrated limbal vessels.[40] IgM predominates in the corneal limbus, being restricted from the central cornea by its large pentameric size. The relative state of hydration of the cornea is thought to influence immunoglobulin diffusion. The immunoglobulins in the cornea, which are cationically charged, are confined to the stromal layers where their binding to proteoglycans and anionic glycosaminoglycans is thought to play a role in regulating their tissue distribution.[41,42] In response to certain antigens placed on the cornea, ring-shaped infiltrates can form in the corneal stroma, which are concentric with the limbus. These rings, referred to as *Wessely rings*, are thought to represent the site of deposition of antigen/antibody complexes. Corneal rings may form in response to corneal gram-negative bacterial infection. In such a case, it has been suggested that the ring that forms actually consists of neutrophils and certain complement proteins, as opposed to antigen/antibody complexes.[43]

Complement proteins are also found in the cornea. These include proteins C1–C7,[44,45] properdin (a stabilizer of C3 convertase), and factor B,[46] as well as the regulatory protein factors H and I, and C1 inhibitor.[47] The trimolecular, high-molecular-weight structure of C1, a critical component in the initiation of the classical pathway of activation, is present in high concentrations in the limbus but is restricted from the central cornea. Its relative abundance in the limbus makes this region particularly susceptible to ulceration after complement activation and immune complex deposition. It is believed that although C1 is produced by corneal fibroblasts, all other corneal complement proteins are derived from the plasma by way of the limbal vasculature.[44]

Ocular complement proteins involved in the alternative pathway are believed to play a role in eliminating *Pseudomonas aeruginosa* bacteria, the endotoxin of which activates these proteins.[48] In general terms, however, the relative importance of complement proteins in the protection of the ocular surface from infection is unclear because the rate of ocular infection is not increased in patients with complement disorders.

Conjunctival Immunology

The conjunctiva, together with the gastrointestinal and respiratory tract mucosas, is part of the mucosal immune system. Specifically, mucosal immune constituents in the conjunctiva have been referred to as *conjunctiva-associated lymphatic tissue* (CALT). They include Langerhans' cells and lymphocytes in the conjunctival epithelium, and dendritic cells, lymphocytes, neutrophils, mast cells, IgA, and IgG in the substantia propria. Under normal conditions, eosinophils and basophils are not present in the conjunctiva.

Conjunctival mast cells play an important role in various allergic states, as described in Chapter 4. With regard to the lymphocyte population, T cells generally predominate, with B cells absent and plasma cells present only in the conjunctival accessory lacrimal glands of Krause or minor lacrimal glands.[49]

Langerhans' cells in the epithelium together with dendritic cells in the substantia propria are thought to present antigens, in the context of class II molecules, to conjunctival helper T cells. These cells then secrete a host of cytokines, including the macrophage-activating cytokine IFN-γ that promotes antigen elimination by macrophages. This essentially represents a delayed-type hypersensitivity (DTH) reaction. Small, nodular DTH reactions of the conjunctiva are referred to as *phlyctenules* and often occur near the corneal limbus. Offending antigens that can lead to the formation of phlyctenules include *Staphylococcus* and *Mycobacteria tuberculosis* bacteria, the yeastlike fungus *Candida*, and the protozoan parasite *Coccidioides*.[50] Class I presentation of antigen to cytotoxic T cells also occurs and results in the destruction of infected cells.

The blood vessels of the conjunctiva are fenestrated. Lymphatic vessels in the bulbar conjunctiva exist as two plaits, one superficial and the other deep. A major component of the superficial plexus is an incomplete pericorneal lymphatic ring. The bulbar and palpebral lymphatic vessels ultimately drain into various nodes, including the preauricular, parotid, and submandibular lymph nodes. Thus, the conjunctiva has all the elements required to mediate both the afferent and efferent limbs of an immune response.

Some evidence suggests that human conjunctival epithelial cells secrete proinflammatory cytokines. In their resting state, these cells were shown to secrete IL-1 receptor antagonist.[51] When stimulated, they produced TNF-α, IL-6, IL-8, and granulocyte-monocyte cerebrospinal fluid in a dose- and time-dependent fashion. It therefore seems reasonable to suggest an effector role for these cells in certain cases of ocular inflammation such as allergic and chronic conjunctivitis.[51]

Scleral Immunology

The sclera consists primarily of compact, fibrous connective tissue that is continuous with the corneal stroma. Unlike the cornea, scleral connective tissue contains irregularly arranged collagen fibers, more elastic tissue, blood vessels (not many—the sclera is relatively avascular), and a dearth of acidic mucopolysaccharides.[52] Very few immune cells are found in the sclera. In response to antigenic stimulation, however, immune cells and complement components are recruited into the sclera from the overlying episcleral vessels and underlying choroidal vasculature.[53,54] Complement components that have been detected in the sclera include proteins C1–C6, and factor B.[53] Scleral fibroblasts, like their corneal counterparts, can constitutively express complement protein C1. Recombinant human IFN-γ can increase this production and also induce the formation of proteins C2 and C4.[55] Large amounts of IgG and lesser amounts of IgA are found in the sclera.[56] It is thought that IgM is absent from the sclera because it is too large to fit through the fenestrations of the vessels discussed above.[40]

Uveal Immunology

The uveal tract, comprising the iris, ciliary body, and choroid, is a highly vascular tissue. Many of the vessels in the uvea are fenestrated and play an important role in uveal infection and the immune response to it. In particular, the choroidal blood flow is relatively large and consists of, in part, the choriocapillaris, a sinusoidal system just beneath Bruch's membrane. The endothelial cells lining the choriocapillaris are fenestrated and quite thin on their retinal side, but are thicker and covered by pericytes on their scleral side. Such an arrangement attests to the importance of the choriocapillaris to normal retinal pigment epithelial cell function.

The lobulated arrangement of the extensive choriocapillaris, coupled with its large blood flow, facilitates the trapping of circulating infectious agents, most notably fungi. In fact, most fungal infections cause choroiditis early in their course.[57] Its considerable blood flow also plays an important role in facilitating the transport of immunoreactive cells.[58] The connective tissue stroma of the uveal tract, which normally has a complement of mast cells, macrophages, lymphocytes, and plasma cells, can readily increase its immune cell numbers in infectious or autoimmune states (i.e., uveitis). Although it has been taught that the choroid lacks lymphatic vessels, some data challenge this conclusion.[58]

In addition to the cellular elements of the immune response, the uvea also contains a host of immune factors. In the choroid, moderate amounts of IgG and IgA can be found deposited along anionic sites of Bruch's membrane.[59–61] C3 complement protein was shown to be present in the choroidal stroma and ciliary body, and on Bruch's membrane.[40]

The iris only contains appreciable amounts of IgG and IgA in patients with iritis whose blood/iris barrier has been compromised.[62] The aqueous humor, which has unrestricted access to the iris stroma, contains some IgG and IgA. However, because of the combined circumstances of high aqueous turnover and a lack of anionic sites in the iris that can bind these antibodies, their normal levels in the iris are extremely low.[63]

The ciliary body, which like the choroid has fenestrated vessels, similarly has large amounts of IgG and smaller amounts of IgA.[40] Also as in the choroid, anionic connective tissue elements serve to retain these immunoglobulins for a period of time. C3 complement protein is also present.

Hypersensitivity Reactions in the Uvea

Most cases of ocular inflammation affect the uveal tissues because of their access to the circulation. Such inflammatory reactions are referred to as *uveitis* and can occur in response to infection or autoimmunity, the latter of which is discussed in Chapter 5.

All four types of hypersensitivity reactions are known to occur in the eye. Release of mast cell mediators in the uvea in a type I reaction seems to play a complementary role in the recurrence of uveitis in susceptible individuals during allergy season.[64] These mediators induce the influx of lymphocytes into the uveal connective tissue, resulting in an exacerbation of an underlying episodic uveitic condition. Type II reactions, of which there are four subtypes, are those mediated in one way or another by antibodies. In ocular cicatricial pemphigoid, antibodies directed to basement membrane proteins on the surface of the eye induce scarring. In the uvea, however, it does not appear that such a reaction plays an important role in uveal immunity nor is it of major consequence in uveitis.

A type III reaction, referred to as *immune complex inflammation*, occurs as a result of the deposition of immune complexes. It is clear that many cases of uveitis develop as a result of this type of reaction. The complexes that deposit in the uveal tract induce damage by activating complement, which triggers leukocyte chemotaxis, release of vasoactive amines from mast cells and basophils, increased vascular permeability, platelet aggregation and microthrombus formation, and release of lysosomal enzymes from neutrophils.[40]

Complexes can either form locally in the eye or be deposited there from the vasculature. IgG, IgM, and IgA have all been implicated in complex formation. Various factors play a role in complex deposition, including size, charge, anatomic and hemodynamic factors, and the innate ability to clear complexes. Some of these factors are also important in determining where complexes will accumulate. As mentioned above, cationic immunoglobulins bind to anionic sites in the uveal connective tissue. These trapped antibodies can then form complexes with antigen and cause localized inflammation. Uveal regions that are prone to the development of this type of immune complex inflammation include tissue adjacent to Bruch's membrane in the choroid, and the ciliary process, which is nourished by tortuous blood vessels.[61] On the other hand, circulating immune complexes (i.e., preformed immune complexes) preferentially deposit in the limbal-scleral capillary plexus, with occasional deposits in the iris and choriocapillaris (Figure 3.5).[61,65,66] Immune complex deposition has also been implicated in cases of retinal vasculitis.[67,68]

Type IV, or DTH, reactions are mediated by T cells and macrophages. Contact dermatitis, interstitial keratitis, vernal keratoconjunctivitis, giant papillary conjunctivitis, granulomatous inflammation in sympathetic ophthalmia, Behçet's disease, sarcoidosis, and autoimmune uveitis are all syndromes which result, at least in part, from a DTH reaction to antigen. A more complete discussion of the immunology of these syndromes can be found in Chapters 4 and 5.

Retinal Immunology

The retina is susceptible to autoimmune attack as well as infection, particularly by neurotropic viruses such as *Toxoplasma gondii*. Immune cells, immunoglobulins, and other high-molecular-weight immune system proteins are prevented from entering retinal tissue by the tight junctions linking the endothelial cells of the retinal vasculature (though recent data, discussed in Chapter 2, appear to challenge this notion). All this can

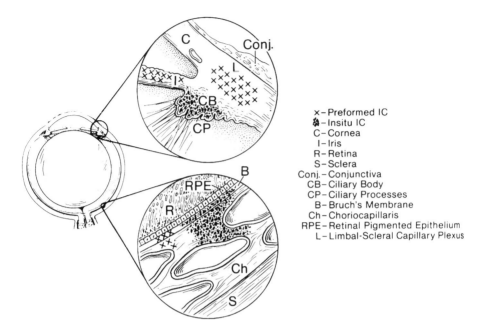

FIGURE 3.5. Schematic representation of the intraocular distribution of in situ immune complexes (ICs) versus preformed ICs. (Reprinted with permission from JC Waldrep, HJ Kaplan, M Warbington. In situ immune complex formation within the uvea. Invest Ophthalmol Vis Sci 1987;28:1191–1195.)

change during inflammation of the neighboring choroid, where factors can be released that can break down this barrier. Indeed, in severe cases of posterior uveitis, immune cells and factors readily enter and destroy retinal tissue. Retinal Müller cells may play a role in downregulating the immune response in the retina, as explained in Chapter 2.

References

1. Stein R, Hurwitz JJ. Anatomy and Physiology of Tear Secretion. In JJ Hurwitz (ed), The Lacrimal System. Philadelphia: Lippincott–Raven, 1996;1.
2. Milder B. The Lacrimal Apparatus. In RA Moses, WM Hart (eds), Adler's Physiology of the Eye: Clinical Applications. St. Louis: Mosby, 1987;15.
3. Sack RA, Tan KO, Tan A. Diurnal tear cycle: evidence for a nocturnal inflammatory constitutive tear fluid. Invest Ophthalmol Vis Sci 1992;33:626–640.
4. Milder B. The Lacrimal Apparatus. In RA Moses, WM Hart (eds), Adler's Physiology of the Eye: Clinical Applications. St. Louis: Mosby, 1987;22.

5. Watanabe H, Tisdale AS, Gipson IK. Eyelid opening induces expression of a glycocalyx glycoprotein on rat ocular surface epithelium. Invest Ophthalmol Vis Sci 1993;34:327–338.

6. Gipson IK, Yankauckas SJ, Spurr-Michaud SJ, et al. Characteristics of a glycoprotein in the ocular surface glycocalyx. Invest Ophthalmol Vis Sci 1992;33: 218–227.

7. Yolken RH, Ojeh C, Khatri IA, et al. Intestinal mucins inhibit rotavirus replication in an oligosaccharide-dependent manner. J Infect Dis 1994;169:1002–1006.

8. Foster CS, Shaw CD, Wells PA. Scanning electron microscopy of conjunctival surfaces in patients with ocular cicatricial pemphigoid. Am J Ophthalmol 1986;102:584–591.

9. Wells PA, Ashur ML, Foster CS. SDS-gradient polyacrylamide gel electrophoresis of individual ocular mucus samples from patients with normal and diseased conjunctiva. Curr Eye Res 1986;5:823–831.

10. Stein R, Hurwitz JJ. Anatomy and Physiology of Tear Secretion. In JJ Hurwitz (ed), The Lacrimal System. Philadelphia: Lippincott–Raven, 1996;4.

11. Brock J. Lactoferrin: a multifunctional immunoregulatory protein? Immunol Today 1995;16:417–419.

12. Kijlstra A, Jeurissen SH. Modulation of classical C_3 convertase of complement by tear lactoferrin. Immunology 1982;47:263–270.

13. Bullen JJ, Rogers HJ, Leigh L. Iron-binding proteins in milk and resistance to *Escherichia coli* infection in infants. BMJ 1972;1:69–75.

14. Jones EM, Smart A, Bloomberg G, et al. Lactoferricin, a new antimicrobial peptide. J Appl Bacteriol 1994;77:208–214.

15. Pietsch RL, Pearlman ME. Human tear lysozyme variables. Arch Ophthalmol 1973;90:94–96.

16. Friedlaender MH. Allergy and Immunology of the Eye (2nd ed). Philadelphia: Raven Press, 1993;53.

17. Benjamini E, Sunshine G, Leskowitz S. Immunology: A Short Course (3rd ed). New York: Wiley, 1996;84.

18. Montgomery PC, Rockey JH, Majumdar AS, et al. Parameters influencing the expression of IgA antibodies in tears. Invest Ophthalmol Vis Sci 1984;25:369–373.

19. O'Sullivan NL, Montgomery PC. Selective interactions of lymphocytes with neonatal and adult lacrimal gland tissues. Invest Ophthalmol Vis Sci 1990;31:1615–1622.

20. Ford LC, DeLange RJ, Petty RW. Identification of a nonlysozymal bactericidal factor (beta lysin) in human tears and aqueous humor. Am J Ophthalmol 1976;81:30–33.

21. Bukharin OV, Suleimanov KG. [The role of the thrombocytic cationic protein (beta lysin) in anti-infectious protection.] Zh Mikrobiol Epidemiol Immunobiol 1997;1:3–6.

22. Willcox MD, Morris CA, Thakur A, et al. Complement and complement regulatory proteins in human tears. Invest Ophthalmol Vis Sci 1997;38:1–8.

23. Carmody PJ, Rattazzi MC, Davidson RG. Tay Sachs disease—the use of tears for the detection of heterozygotes. N Engl J Med 1973;289:1072–1074.

24. Fullard RJ, Snyder C. Protein levels in nonstimulated and stimulated tears of normal human subjects. Invest Ophthalmol Vis Sci 1990;31:1119–1126.

25. Bogart B, Sack RA, Beaton A, et al. SigA glycoproteins and soluble mucin in reflex and closed eye tears: does the epithelium shed its membrane-bound mucin? (abstract). Invest Ophthalmol Vis Sci 1994;35(suppl):1560.

26. Sack RA, Bogart BI, Beaton A, et al. Diurnal variations in tear glycoproteins: evidence for an epithelial origin for the major non-reducible ≥450 kDa sialo-glycoprotein(s). Curr Eye Res 1997;16:577–588.

27. Sack RA, Underwood PA, Tan KO, et al. Vitronectin-possible contribution to the closed-eye external host-defense mechanism. Ocul Immunol Inflamm 1993;1:327–336.

28. Streilein JW, Bradley D, Sano Y, Sonoda Y. Immunosuppressive properties of tissues obtained from eyes with experimentally manipulated corneas. Invest Ophthalmol Vis Sci 1996;37:413–424.

29. Bouchard CS. The Ocular Immune Response. In JH Krachmer, MJ Mannis, EJ Hollands (eds), Cornea: Fundamentals of Cornea and External Disease. St. Louis: Mosby, 1997;101.

30. Donnelly JJ, Chan LS, Xi MS, Rockey JH. Effect of human corneal fibroblasts on lymphocyte proliferation in vitro. Exp Eye Res 1988;47:61–70.

31. Cubitt CL, Lausch RN, Oakes JE. Differences in interleukin-6 gene expression between cultured human corneal epithelial cells and keratocytes. Invest Ophthalmol Vis Sci 1995;36:330–336.

32. Elner VM, Strieter RM, Pavilack MA, et al. Human corneal interleukin-8. IL-1 and TNF-induced gene expression and secretion. Am J Pathol 1991; 139:977–988.

33. Niederkorn JY, Peeler JS, Mellon J. Phagocytosis of particulate antigens by corneal epithelial cells stimulates interleukin-1 secretion and migration of Langerhans' cells into the central cornea. Reg Immunol 1989;2:83–90.

34. Chandler, JW. Ocular Surface Immunology. In JS Pepose, GN Holland, KR Wilhelmus (eds), Ocular Infection and Immunity. St. Louis: Mosby, 1996;104–111.

35. Roussel TJ, Osato MS, Wilhelmus KR. Corneal Langerhans' cell migration following ocular contact sensitivity. Cornea 1983;2:27–30.

36. Sano Y, Streilein JW. Effects of Corneal Surgical Wounds on Ocular Immune Privilege. In RB Nussenblatt, SM Whitcup, RR Caspi, I Gery (eds), Advances in Ocular Immunology. Bethesda, MD: Elsevier Science BV, 1994;207–210.

37. Elner VM, Elner SG, Pavilack MA, et al. Intercellular adhesion molecule-1 in human corneal endothelium. Modulation and function. Am J Pathol 1991;138:525–536.

38. Foets BJ, van den Oord JJ, Volpes R, Missotten L. In situ immunohistochemical analysis of cell adhesion molecules on human corneal endothelial cells. Br J Ophthalmol 1992;76:205–209.

39. Iwata M, Yagihashi A, Roat MI, et al. Human leukocyte antigen-class II-positive human corneal epithelial cells activate allogeneic T cells. Invest Ophthalmol Vis Sci 1994;35:3991–4000.

40. Waldrep JC, Mondino BJ. Humoral Immunity and the Eye. In JS Pepose, GN Holland, KR Wilhelmus (eds), Ocular Infection and Immunity. St. Louis: Mosby, 1996;33–49.

41. Waldrep JC. Uveal IgG distribution: regulation by electrostatic interactions. Curr Eye Res 1987;6:897–907.

42. Waldrep JC, Noe RL, Stulting RD. Analysis of human corneal IgG by isoelectric focusing. Invest Ophthalmol Vis Sci 1988;29:1538–1543.

43. Mondino BJ, Rabin BS, Kessler E, et al. Corneal rings with gram-negative bacteria. Arch Ophthalmol 1977;95:2222–2225.

44. Mondino BJ. Studies of Complement in Corneal Tissue. In GR O'Connor, JW Chandler (eds), Advances in Immunology and Immunopathology of the Eye. New York: Masson, 1985;194–198.

45. Mondino BJ, Hoffman DB. Hemolytic complement activity in normal human donor corneas. Arch Ophthalmol 1980;98:2041–2044.

46. Mondino BJ, Ratajczak HV, Goldberg DB, et al. Alternate and classical pathway components of complement in the normal cornea. Arch Ophthalmol 1980;98:346–349.

47. Mondino BJ, Sumner H. Complement inhibitors in normal cornea and aqueous humor. Invest Ophthalmol Vis Sci 1984;25:483–486.

48. Holland GN, Pepose JS, Dinning WJ. Ophthalmic Disorders Associated with Selected Primary and Acquired Immunodeficiency Diseases. In W Tasman, EA Jaeger (eds), Duane's Clinical Ophthalmology, vol. 5. Philadelphia: Lippincott–Raven, 1996;1–20.

49. Sacks EH, Wieczorek R, Jakobiec FA, Knowles DM II. Lymphocytic subpopulations in the normal human conjunctiva. A monoclonal antibody study. Ophthalmology 1986;93:1276–1283.

50. Friedlaender MH. Allergy and Immunology of the Eye (2nd ed). Philadelphia: Raven Press, 1993;59.

51. Gamache DA, Dimitrijevich SD, Weimer LK, et al. Secretion of proinflammatory cytokines by human conjunctival epithelial cells. Recept Signal Transduct 1997;5:117–128.

52. Kuwabara T. The Eye. In L Weiss (ed), Cell and Tissue Biology: A Textbook of Histology (5th ed). Baltimore: Urban and Schwarzenberg, 1983;1082.

53. Brawman-Mintzer O, Mondino BJ, Mayer FJ. Distribution of complement in the sclera. Invest Ophthalmol Vis Sci 1989;30:2240–2244.

54. Fong LP, Sainz de la Maza M, Rice BA, et al. Immunopathology of scleritis. Ophthalmology 1991;98:472–479.

55. Harrison SA, Mondino BJ, Mayer FJ. Scleral fibroblasts. Human leukocyte antigen expression and complement production. Invest Ophthalmol Vis Sci 1990;31:2412–2419.

56. Allansmith MR, Whitney CR, McClellan BH, Newman LP. Immunoglobulins in the human eye: location, type, and amount. Arch Ophthalmol 1973;89:36–45.

57. Cogan DG. Immunosuppression and eye disease. Am J Ophthalmol 1977;83:777–788.

58. Junghans BM, Crewther SG, Crewther DP, Pirie B. Lymphatic sinusoids exist in chick but not in rabbit choroid. Aust N Z J Ophthalmol 1997;25(suppl 1):103–105.

59. Peress NS, Tompkins DC. Pericapillary permeability of the ciliary processes: role of molecular charge. Invest Ophthalmol Vis Sci 1982;23:168–175.

60. Pino RM, Essner E, Pino LC. Location and chemical composition of anionic sites in Bruch's membrane of the rat. J Histochem Cytochem 1982;30:245–252.

61. Waldrep JC, Kaplan HJ, Warbington M. In situ complex formation within the uvea. Potential role of cationic antibody. Invest Ophthalmol Vis Sci 1987;28:1191–1195.

62. Ghose T, Quigley JH, Landrigan PL, Asif A. Immunoglobulins in aqueous humour and iris from patients with endogenous uveitis and patients with cataract. Br J Ophthalmol 1973;57:897–903.

63. Baba H. Histochemical and polarization optical investigation for glycosaminoglycans in exfoliation syndrome. Graefes Arch Clin Exp Ophthalmol 1983;221:106–109.

64. Ruedemann AD. Ocular Manifestations of Allergy. In JW Thomas (ed), Allergy in Clinical Practice. Philadelphia: Lippincott, 1961;256–274.

65. Hylkema HA, Broersma L, Kijlstra A. In vivo and in vitro deposition of immunoglobulin aggregates in the mouse eye. Curr Eye Res 1988;7:593–599.

66. Hylkema HA, Rathman WM, Kijlstra A. Deposition of immune complexes in the mouse eye. Exp Eye Res 1983;37:257–265.

67. Andrews BS, McIntosh J, Petts V, Penny R. Circulating immune complexes in retinal vasculitis. Clin Exp Immunol 1977;29:23–29.

68. Kasp-Grochowska E, Graham E, Sanders MD, et al. Autoimmunity and circulating immune complexes in retinal vasculitis. Trans Ophthalmol Soc UK 1981;101(pt 3):342–348.

CHAPTER 4

The Ocular Allergic Response

The result of these experiments so far is to show that the morbidity of hay fever patients may be decreased, by properly injected dosage, at least a hundredfold, while excessive or too frequent inoculations only serve to increase the sensibility.*

Adaptive immune responses are characterized by their antigen specificity and by their ability to exhibit enhanced responsiveness on secondary exposure to antigen (i.e., memory). When a secondary response occurs in an exaggerated or inappropriate way, the condition is referred to as *hypersensitivity*. Although the term *allergy* was originally defined as altered immune reactivity on second contact with antigen, it now generally refers to a type I hypersensitivity reaction. Some of the more severe ocular allergies are manifestations of both type I and type IV reactions. Ten percent to 20% of the population has allergies; of these individuals, more than one-third have ocular manifestations. Most develop their allergy during childhood, and there appears to be a genetic link related to total immunoglobulin E (IgE) levels and enhanced immune responsiveness. Fortunately, many have only mild ocular involvement and respond well to over-the-counter or prescription drugs for relief of their ocular inflammation and itching (the cardinal symptom). An important group, however, experiences significant corneal pathology and ocular morbidity.[1]

This chapter describes the four classic forms of ocular allergy and discusses some of the therapeutic approaches being used to treat them. The four conditions are seasonal allergic conjunctivitis (SAC), vernal keratoconjunctivitis (VKC), giant papillary conjunctivitis (GPC), and atopic keratoconjunctivitis. Because all of these conditions are examples of type I or type

---

*From the first reported use of desensitization therapy for the treatment of hay fever, by L Noon, BC Cantab, *The Lancet* 1911.

I and type IV hypersensitivity reactions, we begin with a brief review of the mechanism of these reactions and then provide a description of the clinical tests used to assess allergy.

Review of Type I and Type IV Hypersensitivity Reactions

Type I, or immediate, hypersensitivity is triggered by secondary exposure to environmental antigens such as pollens (tree and grass), mold spores, feces of dust mites, and animal dander. In this context, these antigens are referred to as *allergens*. When initially exposed to allergens, a sensitive individual will respond by producing IgM antibodies. In response to T cell–derived interleukin-4 (IL-4), a switch to the IgE isotype occurs. IgE then binds by its Fc region to a receptor on the surface of mast cells. On re-exposure, the allergen binds to the Fab region of mast cell–bound IgE, cross-linking adjacent molecules and quickly leading to the activation of protein kinase C. This enzyme phosphorylates myosin light chains and leads to the disassembly of actin-myosin complexes beneath the plasma membrane, clearing the way for the release of mast cell granules containing histamine and heparin.

Allergen re-exposure also activates the rate-limiting enzyme phospholipase A_2 both directly and indirectly through an induced elevation of intracellular Ca^{++}, which catalyzes the liberation of membrane arachidonic acid. Under the influence of lipoxygenase, cyclooxygenase, and acetyl transferase enzymes, arachidonic acid is then converted into leukotrienes (LTB_4, LTC_4, LTD_4, and LTE_4), prostaglandins (PGD_2), and platelet-activating factor (PAF), respectively. Collectively, the preformed and newly formed mediators act as chemoattractants and vasodilators and also increase vascular permeability and induce bronchial constriction.

Mast cells also release various cytokines such as tumor necrosis factor and IL-1, which, together with IL-5 released from Th2 cells, are thought to play a role in triggering the late phase of the type I reaction that occurs after several hours. These cytokines have been implicated in the recruitment of eosinophils, basophils, and Th2 cells into the site of antigen exposure. An example of a late-phase reaction is eczema or atopic dermatitis.

In a type IV, or delayed-type hypersensitivity (DTH) reaction, Langerhans' cells present epitopes of the allergen to T cells, which secrete cytokines that recruit mononuclear cells and macrophages and activate them to remove the stimulating allergen. Unlike immediate hypersensitivity, which occurs within minutes and is mediated by antibody, the DTH reaction occurs over 2–3 days and is cell mediated. The three types of DTH are contact hypersensitivity, the tuberculin reaction, and granulomatous inflammation. For a more complete description of all of the above reactions, please refer to Chapter 1.

Tests to Define Clinical Allergy
(Type I Hypersensitivity)

When intradermally challenged with an allergen, a sensitive individual will exhibit a classical wheal and flare reaction characterized by an area of edema surrounded by an area of erythema. The degree of reactivity is usually concentration dependent. In a test called the *Prausnitz-Kustner test*, the presence of reactive IgE can be demonstrated by injecting the individual's serum into a normal subject or animal and challenging the recipient a day or two later with intradermal antigen. The presence of allergen-specific IgE can also be demonstrated in vitro using the *radioallergosorbent test*. In this test, the allergen is linked to an immunoabsorbent paper disk that is treated with the patient's serum. The amount of bound IgE is then determined by the addition of labeled anti-IgE antibodies.

Seasonal Allergic Conjunctivitis

Clinical Features

Seasonal allergens such as pollens, grasses, and outdoor molds, and perennial allergens such as dust mites, indoor molds, and animal dander can all precipitate an immediate hypersensitivity reaction in the nasal mucosa and ocular tissues.[2] Ocular symptoms include itching (ocular and periocular), tearing, burning, pressure behind the eyes, stinging, and photophobia.[3] Ocular symptoms directly correlate with the degree of allergen exposure, and in the case of seasonal allergens, wax and wane with the rise and fall of airborne pollens. In general, allergy sufferers tend to do worse in warm, dry climates and better in cooler, more humid climates.

The classic clinical signs of SAC are an edematous (chemotic) and hyperemic conjunctiva, lid and periorbital swelling, excess lacrimation, and watery discharge (Color Plate III). Edema in the periorbital tissues may be so acute as to impede blood flow through the periorbital veins, resulting in a deepening of the periorbital skin color called an *allergic shiner*.

Pathogenesis

SAC is a classic example of a type I hypersensitivity reaction. As in skin and mucosal type I reactions, the ocular manifestations occur within minutes but also have a second phase that begins several hours later. Initial allergen-induced production of IgE occurs in B cells, resulting in an elevation in serum and tear fluid levels of the antibody. Allergen-specific IgE in tears seems to be produced locally and is not simply exudated from plasma.[4] There is a high correlation between symptoms of ocular allergy and the presence of allergen-specific IgE in tears, but only a poor correlation was found with specific and/or total IgE in sera.[4] Release of IL-4 from helper T cells plays an important role in the production of IgE,[5] as mentioned earlier. In fact, transgenic animals that overexpress this cytokine were shown to develop an allergic inflammatory disease.[6] IgE then binds to, and "arms," mast cells in the substantia propria of the conjunctiva by way of high affinity Fc receptors. On allergen re-exposure, surface IgE cross-linking occurs, resulting in the release of a host of mast cell mediators, most notably histamine, tryptase, PAF, prostaglandins, leukotrienes, and several eosinophil-derived factors, such as eosinophil chemotactic factor.[7]

Histamine

Histamine mediates ocular itching and hyperemia by binding to H_1 and H_2 receptors, respectively.[8,9] Although histamine is normally present in tear fluid at concentrations of 5–10 ng/ml, levels were shown to be markedly elevated (to approximately 16 ng/ml) in allergy patients.[10] Histamine causes endothelial cells to contract, resulting in leakage of plasma from the vasculature, and induces these cells to produce the vasodilators prostacyclin and nitric oxide. Other effects include constriction of bronchial and intestinal smooth muscle.

Tryptase

Tryptase is a major protein in human lung mucosal mast cells that is also present in connective tissue mast cells. This enzyme can directly activate the complement protein, C3, resulting in the production of C3a, which is an anaphylatoxin (this function is inhibited by heparin). As with histamine, increased levels of tryptase were demonstrated in the tear fluid of allergy patients.[2,11] Furthermore, levels were shown to rise in patients after rubbing of the eyes. It was speculated that the ability of tryptase to degrade the bronchodilator vasoactive intestinal polypeptide in the lung could contribute to the action of this enzyme as a bronchoconstrictor.[12]

Mast Cell Mediators Derived
from Membrane Phospholipids

There are three classes of mast cell mediators, PAF, prostaglandins, and leukotrienes, which are not stored in mast cell granules but whose production is initiated by the action of phospholipase A_2 on membrane phospholipids. PAF is produced by acylation of lysoglyceryl ether phosphorylcholine, which is derived from a membrane phospholipid following the action of phospholipase A_2.[13] The prostaglandins and leukotrienes are produced by the action of cyclooxygenase and lipoxygenase enzymes, respectively, on membrane-derived arachidonic acid.

    In addition to its ability to cause platelet aggregation, PAF causes retraction of endothelial cells and relaxation of vascular smooth muscle,

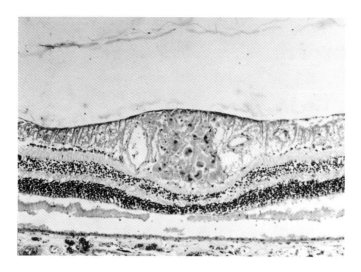

COLOR PLATE I. Section through the retina in the area of a cotton-wool spot showing a cytoid body in the nerve fiber layer. These eosinophilic hyaline structures average 50 mm in diameter with a poorly defined dense core. (Reprinted with permission from U De Girolami, et al. Neuropathology and Ophthalmologic Pathology of Acquired Immunodeficiency Syndrome. Boston: Butterworth–Heinemann, 1992;130.)

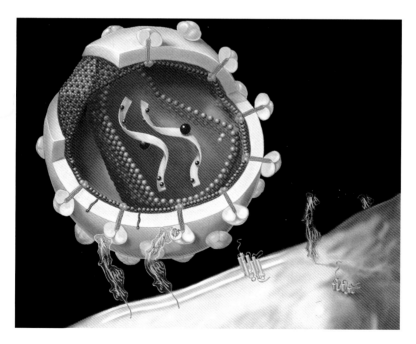

COLOR PLATE II. Structure of the human immunodeficiency virus as depicted adjacent to the surface of a CD4[+] T cell. (Reprinted with permission from front cover, The new face of AIDS. Science 1996;272:1841–2012. Copyright Terese Winslow.)

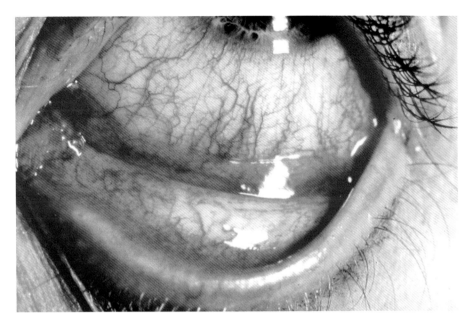

COLOR PLATE III. Seasonal allergy conjunctivitis. Note hyperemic conjunctiva and watery discharge.

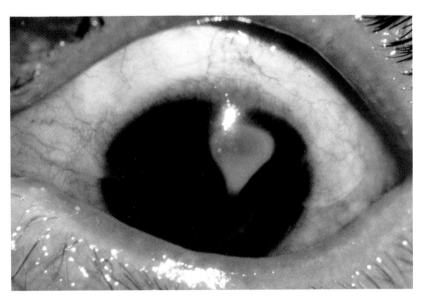

COLOR PLATE IV. Shield ulcer in the superior cornea of a patient with vernal keratoconjunctivitis.

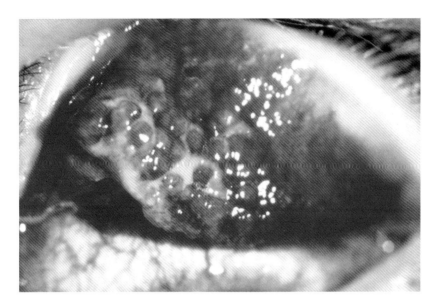

COLOR PLATE V. Giant papillae laced with mucus on the upper tarsal conjunctiva in a patient with giant papillary conjunctivitis.

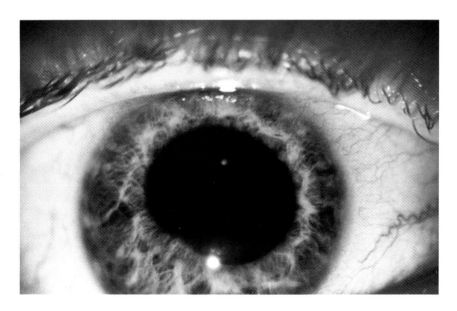

COLOR PLATE VI. Posterior synechia in a patient with uveitis.

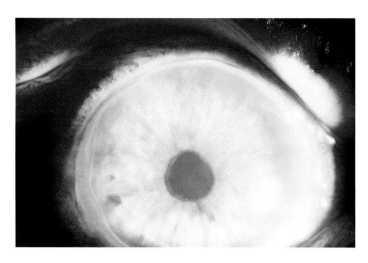

COLOR PLATE VII.   Mooren's ulcer. (Reprinted with permission from MJ Mannis, SM Nagy, M Gershwin. Clinical Allergy Series, Part XI: Allergic and Immunologic Diseases of the Eye. Cypress, CA: Medcom, 1983.)

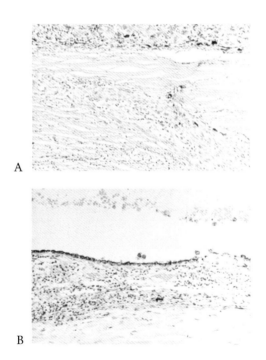

COLOR PLATE VIII.   Histopathology of sympathetic ophthalmia. (A) The choroid is thickened by a granulomatous inflammation in which pale regions represent epithelioid cell formation and dark areas represent regions of lymphocyte accumulation. Sparing of the choriocapillaris and pigment phagocytosis by epithelioid cells is also seen. Note the granulomatous inflammatory involvement of a scleral canal in the lower right corner of the picture. (B) A Dalen-Fuchs nodule representing epithelioid cells between the pigment epithelium and Bruch's membrane. (Reprinted with permission from M Yanoff. Ocular Pathology: A Color Atlas. London: Gower Medical Publishing, 1992;26. By permission of Mosby International.)

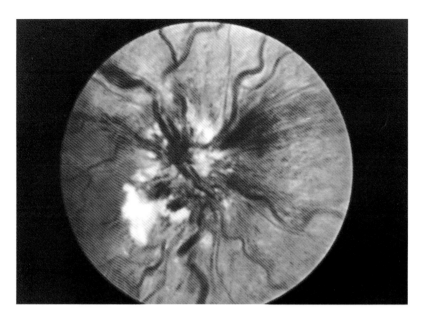

COLOR PLATE IX. Retina of a patient with systemic lupus erythematosus. Note vessel tortuosity, cotton-wool spots, hemorrhages, and edema.

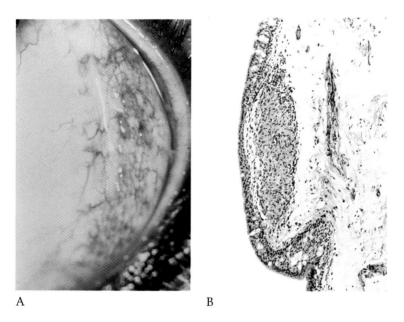

A   B

COLOR PLATE X. Sarcoidosis. (A) Note numerous small, round, translucent cysts in the conjunctival fornix. (B) Conjunctival biopsy revealed a discrete granuloma surrounded by a rim of lymphocytes and plasma cells. (Reprinted with permission from M Yanoff. Ocular Pathology: A Color Atlas. London: Gower Medical Publishing, 1992;30. By permission of Mosby International.)

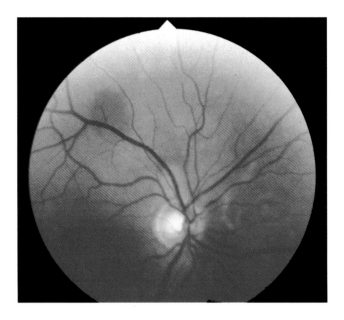

COLOR PLATE XI. Benign choroidal nevus. (Courtesy of Bina Patel, O.D.)

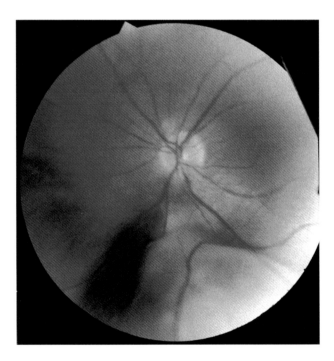

COLOR PLATE XII. Choroidal melanoma with a nonrhegmatous retinal detachment. Ultrasound revealed it to be 8 dd in size. (Courtesy of Bina Patel, O.D.)

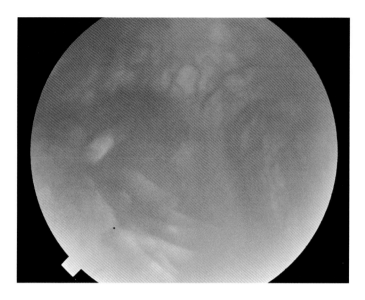

COLOR PLATE XIII.   Diffuse choroidal melanoma.

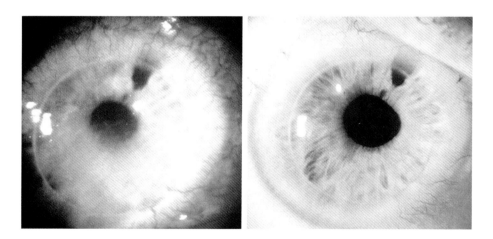

COLOR PLATE XIV.   Corneal allograft endothelial rejection. (Reprinted with permission from JH Krachmer, DA Palay. Corneal Color Atlas. St. Louis: Mosby, 1995.)

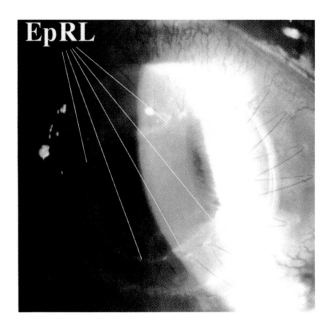

COLOR PLATE XV.   Corneal allograft epithelial rejection. (Reprinted with permission from JH Krachmer, DA Palay. Corneal Color Atlas. St. Louis: Mosby, 1995.)

resulting in increased vascular permeability. It also causes bronchoconstriction and acts as a chemotactic factor for eosinophils and neutrophils. PAF released by vascular endothelial cells rather than by mast cells may be particularly important in the late phase of immediate hypersensitivity because it activates inflammatory leukocytes.[13]

PAF has been shown to act as a chemotactic agent for neutrophils and eosinophils in the conjunctiva and has induced hyperemia and chemosis on exposure in humans and rabbits.[2,14] PAF was also shown to accumulate in the cornea following injury, where it stimulates metalloproteinase gene expression in the epithelium, implicating the factor in extracellular matrix remodeling in wound healing and ulceration.[15] This role of PAF was supported by studies showing release of PAF by UVC-irradiated corneal stromal cells.[16]

Prostaglandins exist in several different forms, some of which have opposing effects. They are found in a host of different tissues and cause peripheral vasodilation, bronchoconstriction, uterine and intestinal smooth muscle contraction, coronary and pulmonary vasoconstriction, inhibition of platelet aggregation, and enhancement of pain-receptor sensitivity. Of the many classes of prostaglandins, it is PGD_2 that is primarily produced by mast cells during the allergic response[17] and induces redness, chemosis, mucous discharge, and a localized eosinophilia when applied to human and guinea pig eyes.[2] Interestingly, nitric oxide and PGE_2 were shown to be produced simultaneously in the conjunctiva during experimentally induced allergic conjunctivitis in guinea pigs.[18] Treatment of these animals with an inhibitor of nitric oxide synthetase reduced the effects of PGD_2, suggesting that nitric oxide may play a role not only in stimulating prostaglandin release but also by acting as a secondary mediator in prostaglandin-induced conjunctival edema. Together with PGE_1, PGE_2, $PGF_{2-\alpha}$, it was shown to be present in ocular tissues and aqueous humor,[2] and the prostaglandin transporter implicated in its uptake and degradation was found to be widely expressed in human ocular tissues.[19]

PGD_2, PGE_2, and PGF are all present in tear fluid.[7,20–22] Although PGE_2 levels do not correlate with clinical signs of inflammation, PGF levels are significantly increased in patients with acute vernal conjunctivitis and chronic trachoma, and PGD_2 levels are increased in tears of allergic patients following conjunctival provocation.

Leukotrienes are produced by the action of lipoxygenase on membrane-derived arachidonic acid. Mast cells primarily produce leukotrienes LTC_4, LTD_4, and LTE_4. These three leukotrienes comprise what was formerly referred to as *slow-reacting substance of anaphylaxis*. Collectively, these substances increase vascular permeability, increase bronchial mucous production, are bronchoconstrictive, and are also chemotactic, chemokinetic, or both. Leukotrienes have been reported to be present in normal tear fluid and in tears after allergen challenge,[23] and levels of LTB_4 were found to be increased in conjunctivitis.[24] LTB_4 was also shown to induce allergic symptoms when topically applied to the surface of the eye, though its effects, ranging from chemosis and vasodilation to eosinophil and neutrophil chemotaxis, varied with species.[25,26] LTC_4 had no effect when topically applied to human and rabbit eyes.[27]

LTB_4 was shown to be one of the major eosinophil chemotactic factors released by mast cells.[28,29] This finding, together with the estimates that half of all patients with SAC exhibit an eosinophilia in their conjunctiva (which is usually free of these cells), has implicated eosinophil-released proteins in the symptomatology of SAC. The appearance of eosinophils is a hallmark of the late phase of SAC.[30] Eosinophils release several proteins, including major basic protein (MBP), eosinophil peroxidase, eosinophil cationic protein (ECP), and eosinophil-derived neurotoxin (EDN). All but EDN are toxic to corneal epithelial cells.[31] MBP comprises nearly half of the protein secreted by eosinophils and is toxic to parasitic larvae such as *Schistosoma mansoni* and *Trichinella spiralis*. Recall that eosinophils play a dominant role in the immune response to parasitic infection.

MBP plays a role in the more severe cases of vernal keratoconjunctivitis and giant papillary conjunctivitis and is discussed below. Release of ECP in the late-phase allergic response relates to the magnitude of the clinical reaction,[30] and levels also rise in the serum[32] and tears[33] of these patients.

Chemokines

Chemokines are structurally homologous cytokines approximately 10 kD in size that have the ability to stimulate chemokinesis and chemotaxis. Two major classes of chemokines exist—one produced by mononuclear cells and the other produced by T cells. It has been speculated that a number of chemokines contribute to the late phase of the allergic response. Accordingly, the injection of chemokines in mice elicited a response reminiscent of the late-phase response.[34] The eosinophil and basophil chemotactic chemokine RANTES (regulated on activation, normal T expressed and secreted) has also been implicated in the allergic response, though interestingly, this chemokine was also suggested to be the histamine release inhibitory factor.[35]

Adhesion Molecules and Cytokines

Adhesion molecules and cytokines have also been implicated in allergic inflammation. Intercellular adhesion molecule–1 (ICAM-1) was shown to be expressed on endothelial cells in the early phase of the allergic response; this expression was blocked by the steroid deflazacort.[36] ICAM-1 was also shown to be expressed on conjunctival epithelial cells in allergic but not nonallergic individuals.[37] As mentioned, IL-4 is also implicated in the allergic response. T cells from patients with conjunctivitis release IL-4 when stimulated in vitro,[38] and increased transcripts of this cytokine, as well as IL-13, a cytokine suggested to play a role in the prolonged release of IgE in allergic disease, were recovered from the conjunctiva of allergy patients.[39]

Vernal Keratoconjunctivitis

VKC is a bilateral and chronic inflammatory disease of the conjunctiva and cornea. It generally afflicts individuals under 30 years old with most patients being adolescents,[40] and more men than women are affected.[41] It develops more frequently in individuals with a family history of atopy and allergic disease, primarily during the spring and summer months. VKC is common in regions where the climate is hot and dry, such as the south-western United States, the Middle East, and portions of Mexico, Africa, and the Indian subcontinent. By comparison, the incidence is low (1 in 5,000 cases of eye disease) in Northern Europe and most of North America.[40]

Clinical Features

VKC can present in two conjunctival forms, palpebral or limbal. The palpebral form is characterized initially by a thickening of the tarsal conjunctiva, which ultimately develops into giant cobblestone papillae that may reach 7–8 mm across.[1] It is easy to understand how such papillae can contribute to the foreign-body sensation that these patients experience. By their sheer weight, these papillae can cause ptosis. In the limbal form, vascularized gelatinous-appearing papillae containing eosinophils, mast cells, lymphocytes, and plasma cells, all in an edematous milieu, form on the bulbar conjunctiva at the corneal limbus, especially superiorly.[41] Characteristic white dots, referred to as *Horner-Trantas dots*, are seen on the limbus within the papillae, which represent degenerating eosinophils and epithelial cells. The limbal form of the disease is more common in darker skinned individuals who live in warm, dry climates.[41,42]

Patients complain first and foremost of itching as well as mucous discharge and tearing. They produce a tough and ropy mucous that insinuates itself between the papillae and may form a pseudomembrane, the *Maxwell-Lyons sign*. Frank corneal involvement may occur and indicates an elevated level of disease severity. Superficial epithelial keratitis may occur, ultimately resulting in the development of "shield ulcers," most often in the superior cornea (Color Plate IV). These ulcers, which can lead to corneal scarring or become sights of microbial infection, are thought to represent the consequence of the toxic action of factors such as eosinophil-derived MBP on the corneal epithelial cells.

Pathogenesis

Types I and IV hypersensitivity contribute to the symptomatology and pathogenesis of VKC. Evidence for type I involvement includes the demonstration of increased numbers of degranulated conjunctival mast cells[43,44] and elevated levels of tryptase, histamine, and IgE, and decreased levels of histaminase in the tear fluid of afflicted individuals.[43,45,46] Eosinophils were also shown to be present in high numbers in the conjunctiva and in Horner-Trantas dots, and, as mentioned, eosinophil-derived factors contribute to corneal ulceration in severe cases.[47] Type IV hypersensitivity was also implicated in this disease by the demonstration of activated (as determined by their expression of IL-2 receptors) CD4+ helper T cells, as well as macrophages in affected eyes.[40,48] These T cells were shown to release cytokines such as IL-3, IL-4, IL-5, and others,[49] which play a role in activating eosinophils and mast cells, as well as increasing class II expression on the conjunctival epithelial and stromal cells, perhaps making the latter cells sensitive to immune-mediated destruction. It has been suggested that VKC represents a phenotypic model of upregulation of a cytokine gene cluster encoding IL-3, IL-4, IL-5, and granulocyte/macrophage-colony–stimulating factor, secretion of which favors Th2 cell activity resulting in IgE production and mast cell and eosinophil activation.[50] The expression of the adhesion molecules ICAM-1, ELAM-1 (endothelial leukocyte adhesion molecule–1), and VCAM-1 (vascular cell adhesion molecule–1) on basal epithelial cells, vascular endothelial cells, or both, was shown to be increased in VKC.[51]

Differential Diagnosis

The condition most closely resembling VKC is AKC. AKC is associated with other manifestations of atopy, such as eczema. As such, patients with AKC tend to experience blepharitis.[40] Furthermore, they experience conjunctival scarring, subepithelial fibrosis, and cicatrization.[40,41] Overall, the lower rather than the upper palpebral conjunctiva is affected in AKC. Finally, AKC patients complain of a watery discharge, not a mucous discharge as seen in VKC.

Because corneal changes are rarely associated with SAC and this condition is also associated with rhinitis and sinusitis, a differential diagnosis with VKC is fairly straightforward.[40] Although the giant papillary reaction in VKC is similar to that seen in GPC, the latter is associated with ocular irritation, most commonly caused by contact lenses; thus, a careful history should assist in making the differential diagnosis. It should be noted that severe cases of VKC—in which patients display Horner-Trantas dots, papillae, and shield ulcers—are quite distinctive and are not easily confused with other conditions.

Giant Papillary Conjunctivitis

GPC represents an allergic response to an irritating antigen, such as contact lenses, ocular prosthesis, protruding corneal sutures, extruded scleral buckles, or other corneal deposits. Specifically, the reaction that occurs in GPC is contact hypersensitivity and as such represents a type IV reaction, though elements of a type I reaction are also seen. Implicit in the fact that this condition represents a reaction to contact with an inducing substance is the notion that GPC, like SAC and VKC, can be alleviated by removal of the offending agent.

Clinical Features

Because GPC occurs most frequently in response to contact lens wear ($\leq 5\%$ of contact lens wearers develop GPC), its clinical features are described with that in mind. Early features of this condition include mild hyperemia and increased mucous coating of the upper tarsal conjunctiva.[52] Patients also complain of itching, which may be severe in later stages. The increased mucous secretion causes excessive movement of the lens during blinking, a condition that rapidly contributes to lens intolerance. As the condition progresses, small papillae form on the tarsal conjunctiva that may ultimately develop in severe cases into the most striking feature of the condition, giant papillae (larger than 1 mm) (Color Plate V). Even when giant papillae are present, some patients may be asymptomatic.[53] In active phases of the disease, there is also tissue edema and cellular infiltration; these, together with the presence of the papillae, may contribute to the development of ptosis. Allansmith has described differential changes in discrete regions of the upper tarsal conjunctiva that occur in response to different types of contact lenses.[52]

Pathogenesis

For many years, it was simply assumed, and data corroborated the assumption, that GPC develops as a result of an immune response to deposits of various materials on the offending contact lens or ocular prosthesis. This was supported by the amelioration of symptoms when a new or cleaned lens was put on the eye. The presence of deposits on lenses, which develop more frequently on high rather than low water content contact lenses,[54] correlated strongly with GPC,[55] and digesting proteinaceous deposits with enzymes increased lens tolerance.[56] Lenses from symptomatic patients also displayed denatured lysozyme and an increase in the IgG to IgA deposition ratio.[57] Lipids on contact lenses do not appear to be antigenic. GPC also occurs, however, as a result of mechanical trauma induced by blinking thousands of times a day over a presumably nonantigenic scleral buckle or corneal protrusion.

Various histopathologic features of GPC suggest the involvement of both types I and IV hypersensitivity reactions in its pathogenesis. Type I involvement is supported by the presence of degranulated mast cells, as well as some eosinophils in the conjunctiva and increased levels of IgE in tear fluid.[53] It has been shown that detecting the leukotriene LTC_4 levels in contact lens wearers can give useful information regarding the presence of contact lens–related subclinical inflammation and subclinical GPC.[58] Type IV involvement is supported by the demonstration of activated, memory CD4+ helper T cells[59] and increased expression of ICAM-1 and other adhesion molecules in the conjunctiva.[53]

Differential Diagnosis

Unlike VKC and AKC, there is no corneal involvement in GPC. Even though the giant papillary reaction in VKC is similar to that seen in GPC, the latter is associated with ocular irritation, most commonly caused by contact lenses; thus, a careful history should assist in making the differential diagnosis. Although microbial conjunctivitis also produces an exudate, it is purulent rather than white and stringy.[53]

Atopic Keratoconjunctivitis

Ocular involvement occurs in up to 40% of patients with a history of atopic dermatitis (i.e., eczema) and takes the form of AKC.[60] Extraocular manifestations include asthma. In general, more men than women are afflicted, and the disease appears to have a genetic component. Unlike other allergic diseases, AKC does not seem to resolve with increasing age.

Clinical Features

AKC is bilateral and some symptoms (itching, tearing, and mucoid discharge) are similar to those seen in other allergic eye diseases. However, AKC patients uniquely demonstrate scaly, crusty, indurated, and inflamed lids that usually show a mucoid exudate along the margin. If severe, ectropion and epiphora may result.[60] The inner and outer canthi may become macerated from tearing.[61] Such conditions are ripe for lid infection and *Staphylococcus aureus* infections develop in two-thirds of patients.[62] The conjunctiva is hyperemic and may exhibit chemosis as well as papillary hypertrophy of the superior and inferior tarsal regions.[60] As with VKC, the upper tarsal conjunctiva may show giant papillae but, unlike VKC, these are usually scarred with flat tops. Conjunctival scarring, subepithelial fibrosis, and cicatrization can also occur.[40,41]

What makes this condition particularly serious is the fact that most patients exhibit some degree of corneal pathology. Less serious corneal involvement takes the form of punctate epithelial keratitis and intraepithelial microcysts and is found in most patients. Fewer patients exhibit ulcerative keratitis and stromal scars. Patients also have an increased frequency of keratoconus and retinal detachments, presumably induced by prolonged rubbing of the eyes. AKC is usually accompanied by facial dermatitis and marks on the face brought on by scratching may be evident.

Pathogenesis

IgE levels are elevated in patients' tears and serum,[62] and they exhibit abnormally high numbers of mast cells and eosinophils in the conjunctival epithelium and substantia propria.[63] Eosinophil-derived proteins such as MBP and

TABLE 4.1
Differential Diagnosis of Ocular Allergy

Finding	*Seasonal Allergic Conjunctivitis*	*Vernal Keratocon-junctivitis*	*Giant Papillary Conjunctivitis*	*Atopic Keratocon-junctivitis*
Cicatrization	no	no	no	yes
Conjunctival scarring	no	no	no	yes
Corneal involvement	no	yes	no	yes
Discharge	watery	mucous	mucous	watery
Giant papillae	no	yes	yes	yes (flat)
Palpebral involvement	no	upper	upper	lower
Associated dermatitis	no	no	no	yes
Associated with contact lens wear	no	no	yes	no

ECP are thought to play a role in the development of keratopathy. Substantial numbers of T cells, B cells, macrophages, and antigen-presenting cells are also seen in the conjunctiva. Furthermore, there is enhanced expression of MHC class II molecules on conjunctival epithelial and endothelial cells.[60] Thus, AKC appears to involve type I and type IV hypersensitivity.

Differential Diagnosis

Unlike SAC and GPC, the cornea is affected in both VKC and AKC. Early VKC can in fact look very similar to AKC. The giant papillae that develop in AKC are scarred and have flat tops in contrast to those in VKC and GPC. AKC is associated with other manifestations of atopy, such as eczema and blepharitis, whereas these other conditions are not. Furthermore, AKC patients experience conjunctival scarring, subepithelial fibrosis, and cicatrization.[40,41] Overall, the lower rather than upper palpebral conjunctiva is affected in AKC compared with VKC. AKC patients exhibit a watery discharge, not a mucous discharge as seen in VKC (see Table 4.1 for differential diagnosis in ocular allergy).

Therapeutic Options for the Treatment of Ocular Allergy

Antihistamines

Systemic

Systemic antihistamines have met with partial success in the treatment of SAC and have had some benefit when given at bedtime as an adjunct treatment for VKC and AKC.[64] The first-generation drugs have the disadvantage of causing drowsiness. The second-generation agents, such as astemizole (Hismanal), terfenadine (Seldane), and loratadine (Claritin), do not cross the blood-brain barrier and as such are nonsedating. These agents block H_1 histamine receptors and prevent pruritus and lacrimation as well as histamine release. A disadvantage of astemizole is that it requires several days of treatment to reach its maximal effect. Drug interaction effects of terfenadine made this drug the least popular choice of the three and resulted in its removal from the market by the U.S. Food and Drug Administration.

Topical

Several topical H_1 antagonist antihistamines are available for the treatment of SAC, many of which are given in combination with vasoconstrictors and reduce both ocular itching and redness. Examples include naphazoline HCl, 0.05%/antazoline phosphate, 0.5% (Vasocon-A), the former being the vasoconstrictor; and naphazoline HCl, 0.025%/pheniramine maleate, 0.3% (Naphcon-A). The H_1 antagonist, levocabastine (Levsin), which has the benefits of rapid and long duration of action (>4 hours), was shown to be very effective in alleviating SAC.[2,65] A promising anti-H_1 drug is emedastine, which was also shown to have a long duration of action.[66]

Mast Cell Stabilizers

These compounds prevent the release of mediators from mast cells. Several mechanisms have been proposed to explain how these agents work. It was suggested that they blocked calcium fluxes in the mast cells, possibly by increasing the intracellular levels of cyclic adenosine monophosphate, preventing IgE surface cross-linking and stabilizing the cell. The mast cell stabilizer nedocromil sodium was shown to inhibit chloride ion flux in mast cells (as well as in epithelial cells and neurons), which could account for the prevention of mast cell degranulation.[67] Other reported actions of this agent include inhibition of IgE isotype switching[68] and inhibition of immunoglobulin production by B cells.[69] Mast cell stabilizing agents have also been shown to significantly reduce effector cell chemotaxis and activation specifically affecting neutrophils, eosinophils, and monocytes,[70] and to inhibit the release of substance P and other neuropeptides from sensory nerve endings.[71]

Cromolyn Sodium

Cromolyn sodium, or disodium cromoglycate (DSCG), is given topically in a 4% solution in saline (Crolom). It was shown to be very effective in alleviating the symptoms of seasonal allergy.[72] DSCG was also very effective in VKC[73] and GPC,[74] and relieved symptoms in nearly two-thirds of AKC patients.[75]

Nedocromil Sodium

In numerous clinical trials, nedocromil sodium (2% solution; Tilavist) was shown to be as, or more, effective than DSCG in preventing seasonal allergy symptoms.[76–78] Because nedocromil not only prevents the release of histamine but also LTC_4 and PGD_2, particularly from mucosal mast cells, it is also beneficial in the treatment of asthma.[79] Nedocromil, administered four times a day to VKC patients, was effective in eliminating symptoms.[76,80] GPC patients showed significantly less itching and mucous discharge with the drug, though only in the early weeks of treatment, and effects on lens tolerance were inconclusive.[81] The effects of nedocromil in AKC are as yet unreported.

Lodoxamide

Lodoxamide (Alomide), perhaps the most potent of the mast cell stabilizers, is recommended for the treatment of VKC.[2] It was shown to be much more effective than cromolyn sodium in controlling itching, epiphora, and foreign body sensation in patients with VKC,[82] though others have disputed these findings.[83] GPC patients also responded to this drug and did so with a faster onset than with cromolyn.[84] Results are not yet available for the effects of the drug in AKC patients.

Corticosteroids

Corticosteroids have been shown to be effective for the treatment of seasonal allergy, VKC, GPC, and AKC. Because their use is associated with numerous side effects, however, including elevated intraocular pressure, infections, cataracts, and delayed wound healing, their use in nonsight-threatening conditions such as SAC and GPC is contraindicated.[2] These drugs (e.g., 1% prednisolone sodium phosphate) are still used for short courses in VKC patients exhibiting severe symptoms[40] and in AKC patients exhibiting conjunctival inflammation or keratitis.[60]

Nonsteroidal Anti-Inflammatory Drugs

Aspirin, ibuprofen, and indomethacin are all examples of nonsteroidal anti-inflammatory drugs (NSAIDs). These drugs work by blocking the enzyme cyclooxygenase, resulting in a suppression of prostacyclin, thromboxane, and prostaglandin synthesis. Of these NSAIDs, only aspirin was shown to be effective when given orally to patients with ocular allergy,[85] particularly in patients with VKC. Several topical NSAIDs are available for the treatment of ocular allergy, including ketorolac tromethamine (Acular), suprofen (Profenal), and flurbiprofen (Ansaid). Ketorolac was the first NSAID approved for use in ocular allergy. It specifically inhibits prostaglandin synthesis and relieves the symptoms of seasonal allergy.[86] Suprofen is effective for the treatment of VKC and GPC,[87,88] and flurbiprofen is effective in patients with SAC.[89]

Miscellaneous Drugs

Topical cyclosporin A, an immunosuppressive agent that blocks the activation of CD4+ T cells, improved the condition of patients with VKC[90,91] and AKC.[92] HEPP, a synthetic pentapeptide consisting of an amino acid sequence identical to the Fc region of the human IgE molecule, has been shown to be efficacious in SAC.[93] This agent is thought to act by interfering with IgE binding to the surface of mast cells. Topical application of corticosteroid creams (0.5–1.0% hydrocortisone) to the eyelids helps to reduce inflammation in AKC.

Immunotherapy

Noon and Cantab[94] were the first to show that immunotherapy could increase resistance to pollen by a factor of up to 1,000. Today, immunotherapy is a recognized and established ingredient in the management of pollen-induced rhinitis/conjunctivitis[95] and is carried out by administering small but increasing doses of allergens. This treatment is generally reserved for use in individuals who are refractory to treatment with topical or oral medications.

How immunotherapy works is still subject to debate, though it seems to exert its effects on both the immediate and late phases of the type I reaction. Certain consistent changes have been reported, including an increase in allergen-specific IgG (specifically, IgG4)[96] and a decrease in IgE.[97] The IgG4 antibodies are thought to act by binding to the allergen and preventing it from binding to armed mast cells. Immunotherapy was also shown to reduce basophil reactivity and sensitivity to allergens, to inhibit allergen-induced T cell and eosinophil recruitment, and to inhibit eosinophil activation in the target organ. It was suggested that it also induced a shift of CD4+ T cell type from the Th2 cell (which promotes allergy) to the Th1 cell (which releases interferon-gamma [IFN-γ], a known inhibitor of IgE synthesis).[98] A promising approach to immunotherapy is oral tolerance. Preliminary studies suggest that microencapsulated allergens taken by mouth reduce ragweed allergy symptoms.[99] Contraindications for immunotherapy include immunodeficiency, pregnancy, autoimmunity, and the use of beta-blockers.[100]

References

1. Seamone CD, Jackson WB. Allergic Ocular Disease. In IR Schwab (ed), Immunology of the External Eye. In Duane's Ophthalmology. Philadelphia: Lippincott–Raven, 1996;20–33.

2. Reiss J, Abelson MB, George MA, Wedner HJ. Allergic Conjunctivitis. In JS Pepose, GN Holland, KR Wilhelmus (eds), Ocular Infection and Immunity. St. Louis: Mosby, 1996;345.

3. Friedlaender MH. Management of ocular allergy. Ann Allergy Asthma Immunol 1995;75:212–222.

4. Hoffmann-Sommergruber K, Ferreira ED, Ebner C, et al. Detection of allergen-specific IgE in tears of grass pollen-allergic patients with allergic rhinoconjunctivitis. Clin Exp Allergy 1996;26:79–87.

5. Finkelman FD, Holmes J, Katona IM, et al. Lymphokine control of in vivo immunoglobulin isotype selection. Annu Rev Immunol 1990;8:303–333.

6. Teppler RI, Levinson A, Stanger BZ, et al. IL-4 induces allergic-like inflammatory disease and alters T cell development in transgenic mice. Cell 1990; 457–467.

7. Proud D, Sweet J, Stein P, et al. Inflammatory mediator release on conjunctival provocation of allergic subjects with allergen. J Allergy Clin Immunol 1990;85:896–905.

8. Weston JH, Udell IJ, Abelson MB. H_1 receptors in the human ocular surface. Invest Ophthalmol Vis Sci 1981;20(suppl):32.

9. Abelson MB, Udell, IJ. H_2-receptors in the human ocular surface. Arch Ophthalmol 1981;99:302–304.

10. Abelson MB, Baird RS, Allansmith MR. Tear histamine levels in vernal keratoconjunctivitis and other ocular inflammations. Ophthalmology 1980;87:812–814.

11. Butrus SI, Ochsner KI, Abelson MB, Schwartz LB. The level of tryptase in human tears: an indicator of activation of conjunctival mast cells. Ophthalmology 1990;97:1678–1683.

12. Tam EK, Caughey GH. Degradation of airway neuropeptides by human lung tryptase. Am J Respir Cell Mol Biol 1990;3:27–32.

13. Abbas AK, Lichtman AH, Pober JS. Cellular and Molecular Immunology. Philadelphia: Saunders, 1994;288.

14. George MA, Smith LM, Berdy GJ, Abelson MB. Platelet activating factor–induced inflammation following topical ocular challenge. Invest Ophthalmol Vis Sci 1990;31(suppl):63.

15. Bazan NG, Allan G. Signal transduction and gene expression in the eye: a contemporary view of the pro-inflammatory, anti-inflammatory, and modulatory roles of prostaglandins and other bioactive lipids. Surv Ophthalmol 1997;41(suppl 2):S23–S34.

16. Sheng Y, Birkle DL. Release of platelet activating factor (PAF) and eicosanoids in UVC-irradiated corneal stromal cells. Curr Eye Res 1995;14:341–347.

17. Abelson MB, Schaeffer K. Conjunctivitis of allergic origin: immunologic mechanisms and current approaches to therapy. Surv Ophthalmol 1993;38(suppl):S115–S132.

18. Meijer F, Tak C, van Haeringen NJ, Kijlstra A. Interaction between nitric oxide and prostaglandin synthesis in the acute phase of allergic conjunctivitis. Prostaglandins 1996;52:431–446.

19. Schuster VL, Lu R, Coca-Prados M. The prostaglandin transporter is widely expressed in ocular tissues. Surv Ophthalmol 1997;41(suppl 2):S41–S45.

20. Aichane A, Campbell AM, Chanal I, et al. Precision of conjunctival provocation tests in right and left eyes. J Allergy Clin Immunol 1993;92:49–55.

21. Gluud BS, Jensen OL, Krogh E, Birgens HS. Prostaglandin E2 level in tears during postoperative inflammation of the eye. Acta Ophthalmol Scand Suppl (Copenh) 1985;63:375–379.

22. Dhir SP, Garg SK, Sharma YR, Lath NK. Prostaglandins in human tears. Am J Ophthalmol 1979;87:403–404.

23. Bisgaard H, Ford-Hutchinson AW, Charleson S, Tauderf E. Production of leukotrienes in human skin and conjunctival mucosa after specific allergen challenge. Allergy 1985;40:417–423.

24. Nathan H, Naveh N, Meyer E. Levels of prostaglandin E_2 and leukotriene B_4 in tears of vernal conjunctivitis patients during a therapeutic trial with indomethacin. Doc Ophthalmol 1994;85:247–257.

25. Butrus SI, Corey EJ, Weston JH, Abelson MB. The effect of leukotriene B_4 in rabbit and guinea pig eyes (abstract). Invest Ophthalmol Vis Sci 1984;25 (suppl):109.

26. Spada CS, Woodward DF, Hawley SB, Nieves AL. Leukotrienes cause eosinophil emigration into conjunctival tissue. Prostaglandins 1986;31:795–809.

27. Weston JH, Abelson MB. Leukotriene C_4 in rabbit and human eyes (abstract). Invest Ophthalmol Vis Sci 1985;26(suppl):191.

28. Makino S, Fukuda T. Eosinophils and allergy in asthma. Allergy Asthma Proc 1995;16:13–21.

29. Sehmi R, Cromwell O, Taylor GW, Kay AB. Identification of guinea pig eosinophil chemotactic factor of anaphylaxis as leukotriene B_4 and 8(s),15(S)-dihydroxy-5,9,11,13(Z,E,Z,E)-eicosatetraenoic acid. J Immunol 1991;147: 2276–2283.

30. Montan PG, van Hage-Hamsten M, Zetterstrom O. Sustained eosinophil cationic protein release into tears after a single high-dose conjunctival allergen challenge. Clin Exp Allergy 1996;26:1125–1130.

31. Trocme SD, Hallberg CK, Gill KS, et al. Effects of eosinophil granule proteins on human corneal epithelial cell viability and morphology. Invest Ophthalmol Vis Sci 1997;38:593–599.

32. Tomassini M, Magrini L, De Petrillo G, et al. Serum levels of eosinophil cationic protein in allergic diseases and natural allergen exposure. J Allergy Clin Immunol 1996;97:1350–1355.

33. Montan PG, van Hage-Hamsten M. Eosinophil cationic protein in tears in allergic conjunctivitis. Br J Ophthalmol 1996;80:556–560.

34. Alam R, Kumar D, Anderson-Walters D, Forsythe PA. Macrophage inflammatory protein-1 alpha and monocyte chemoattractant peptide-1 elicit immediate and late cutaneous reactions and activate murine mast cells in vivo. J Immunol 1994;152:1298–1303.

35. Alam R, Forsythe PA, Lett-Brown MA, Grant JA. Interleukin-8 and RANTES inhibit basophil histamine release induced with monocyte chemotactic and activating factor/monocyte chemoattractant peptide-1 and histamine releasing factor. Am J Respir Cell Mol Biol 1992;7:427–433.

36. Ciprandi G, Buscaglia S, Pesce GP, et al. Deflazacort protects against late-phase but not early-phase reactions induced by the allergen specific conjunctival provocation test. Allergy 1993;48:421–430.

37. Ciprandi G, Buscaglia S, Pesce GP, et al. Allergic subjects express intercellular adhesion molecule-1 (ICAM-1 or DC54) on epithelial cells of conjunctiva after allergen challenge. J Allergy Clin Immunol 1993;91:783–792.

38. Maggi E, Biswas P, Del Prete G, et al. Accumulation of Th-2-like helper T cells in the conjunctiva of patients with vernal conjunctivitis. J Immunol 1991;146:1169–1174.

39. Fujishima H, Saito I, Takeuchi T, et al. Characterization of cytokine mRNA transcripts in conjunctival cells in patients with allergic conjunctivitis. Invest Ophthalmol Vis Sci 1997;38:1350–1357.

40. Brody JM, Foster CS. Vernal Conjunctivitis. In JS Pepose, GN Holland, KR Wilhelmus (eds), Ocular Infection and Immunity. St. Louis: Mosby, 1996;367.

41. Colby K, Dohlman C. Vernal keratoconjunctivitis. Int Ophthalmol Clin 1996; 36:15–20.

42. Dahan E, Appel R. Vernal keratoconjunctivitis in the black child and its response to therapy. Br J Ophthalmol 1983;67:688–692.

43. Ballow M, Mendelson L. Specific immunoglobulin E antibodies in tear secretions of patients with vernal conjunctivitis. J Allergy Clin Immunol 1980;66:112–115.

44. Allansmith MR, Baird RS, Greiner JV. Vernal conjunctivitis and contact lens-associated giant papillary conjunctivitis compared and contrasted. Am J Ophthalmol 1979;87:544–555.

45. Berdy GJ, Levene RB, Bateman ST, et al. Identification of histaminase activity in human tears after conjunctival antigen challenge. Invest Ophthalmol Vis Sci 1990;31(suppl):65.

46. Buckley RJ. Vernal keratoconjunctivitis. Surv Ophthalmol 1988;28:303–308.

47. Abelson MB, Madiwale N, Weston JH. Conjunctival eosinophils in allergic ocular disease. Arch Ophthalmol 1984;102:555–556.

48. Bhan AK, Fujikawa LS, Foster CS. T cell subsets and Langerhans' cells in normal and diseased conjunctiva. Surv Ophthalmol 1982;94:205–212.

49. Lightman S. Therapeutic considerations: symptoms, cells and mediators. Allergy 1995;50(21 suppl):10–13.

50. Bonini S, Bonini S, Lambiase A, et al. Vernal keratoconjunctivitis: a model of 5q cytokine gene cluster disease. Int Arch Allergy Immunol 1995;107:95–98.

51. Abu El-Asrar AM, Geboes K, Tabbara KF, et al. Immunopathogenesis of vernal keratoconjunctivitis. Bull Soc Belge Ophtalmol 1995;261:15–24.

52. Allansmith MR. Giant papillary conjunctivitis. J Am Optom Assoc 1990; 61(suppl):S42–S46.
53. Buckley RJ, Bacon AS. Giant Papillary Conjunctivitis. In JS Pepose, GN Holland, KR Wilhelmus (eds), Ocular Infection and Immunity. St. Louis: Mosby, 1996;362.
54. Minarik L, Rapp J. Protein deposits on individual hydrophilic contact lenses: effects of water and ionicity. CLAO J 1989;15:185–188.
55. Fowler SA, Korb DR, Finnemore VM, Allansmith MR. Surface deposits on worn hard contact lenses. Arch Ophthalmol 1984;102:757–759.
56. Korb DR, Greiner JV, Finnemore VM, Allansmith MR. Treatment of contact lenses with papain. Increase in wearing time in keratoconic patients with papillary conjunctivitis. Arch Ophthalmol 1983;101:48–50.
57. Meisler DM, Keller WB. Contact lens type, material, and deposits and giant papillary conjunctivitis. CLAO J 1995;21:77–80.
58. Sengor T, Irkec M, Gulen Y, et al. Tear LTC_4 levels in patients with subclinical contact lens related giant papillary conjunctivitis. CLAO J 1995;21:159–162.
59. Ballow M, Donshik PC, Rapacz P, et al. Immune responses in monkeys to lenses from patients with contact lens induced giant papillary conjunctivitis. CLAO J 1989;15:64–70.
60. Liesegang TJ. Atopic Keratoconjunctivitis. In JS Pepose, GN Holland, KR Wilhelmus (eds), Ocular Infection and Immunity. St. Louis: Mosby, 1996;377.
61. Allansmith MR. The Eye and Immunology. St. Louis: Mosby, 1982;115.
62. Tuft SJ, Kemeny M, Dart JKG, Buckley RJ. Clinical features of atopic keratoconjunctivitis. Ophthalmology 1991;98:150–158.
63. Foster CS, Rice BA, Dutt JE. Immunopathology of atopic keratoconjunctivitis. Ophthalmology 1991;98:1190–1191.
64. Buckley RJ. Vernal keratopathy and its management. Trans Ophthalmol Soc UK 1981;101:234–238.
65. Abelson MB, Weintraub D. Levocabastine eye drops: a new approach for the treatment of acute allergic conjunctivitis. Eur J Ophthalmol 1994;4:91–101.
66. Sharif NA, Su SX, Yanni JM. Emedastine: a potent, high affinity histamine H_1-receptor-selective antagonist for ocular use: receptor binding and second messenger studies. J Ocul Pharmacol 1994;10:653–664.
67. Alton EW, Norris AA. Chloride transport and the actions of nedocromil sodium and cromolyn sodium in asthma. J Allergy Clin Immunol 1996;98: S102–S106.
68. Loh RK, Jabara HH, Geha RS. Mechanisms of inhibition of IgE synthesis by nedocromil sodium: nedocromil sodium inhibits deletional switch recombination in human B cells. J Allergy Clin Immunol 1996;5:1141–1150.
69. Kimata H, Fujimoto M, Mikawa H. Nedocromil sodium acts directly on human B cells to inhibit immunoglobulin production without affecting cell growth. Immunology 1994;81:47–52.
70. Bruijnzeel PLB, Warringa RAJ, Kok PTM, Kreukniet J. Inhibition of neutrophil and eosinophil induced chemotaxis by nedocromil sodium and sodium cromoglycate. Br J Pharmacol 1990;99:798–802.

71. Foreman JC. Substance P and calcitonin gene-regulated peptide: effects on mast cells and in human skin. Int Arch Allergy Appl Immunol 1987;82:366–371.
72. Allansmith MR, Ross RN. Ocular allergy and mast cell stabilizers. Surv Ophthalmol 1986;30:229–244.
73. Foster CS. Evaluation of topical cromolyn sodium in the treatment of vernal keratoconjunctivitis. Ophthalmology 1988;95:194–201.
74. Kruger CJ, Ehrlers WH, Luistro AE, Donshik PC. Treatment of giant papillary conjunctivitis with cromolyn sodium. CLAO J 1992;18:46–48.
75. Jay TL. Clinical features and diagnosis of adult atopic keratoconjunctivitis and the effect of treatment with sodium cromoglycate. Br J Ophthalmol 1981;65:335–340.
76. Kjellman NI, Stevens MT. Clinical experience with Tilavist: an overview of efficacy and safety. Allergy 1995;50(21 suppl):14–22.
77. Moller C, Berg IM, Kjellman M, Stromberg L. Nedocromil sodium 2% eye drops for twice-daily treatment of seasonal allergic conjunctivitis: a Swedish multicentre placebo-controlled study in children allergic to birch pollen. Clin Exp Allergy 1994;24:884–887.
78. Alexander M. Comparative therapeutic studies with Tilavist. Allergy 1995;50 (21 suppl):23–29.
79. Benbow AG, Eady R, Jackson D. The immunopharmacological actions of nedocromil sodium relative to the use of its 2% ophthalmic solution. Eye 1993;7(pt 3 suppl):26–28.
80. el Hennawi M. A double blind placebo controlled group comparative study of ophthalmic sodium cromoglycate and nedocromil sodium in the treatment of vernal keratoconjunctivitis. Br J Ophthalmol 1994;78:365–369.
81. Bailey CS, Buckley RJ. Nedocromil sodium in contact-lens-associated papillary conjunctivitis. Eye 1993;7(pt 3 suppl):29–33.
82. Cladwell DR, Verin P, Hartwich-Young R, et al. Efficacy and safety of lodoxamide 0.1% vs cromolyn sodium 4% in patients with vernal keratoconjunctivitis. Am J Ophthalmol 1992;113:632–637.
83. Lee S, Allard TRFK. Lodoxamide in vernal keratoconjunctivitis. Ann Pharmacol 1996;30:535–537.
84. Fahy GT, Easty DL, Collum LM, et al. Randomised double-masked trial of lodoxamide and sodium cromoglycate in allergic eye disease. A multicentre study. Eur J Ophthalmol 1992;2(3):144–149.
85. Abelson MB, Butrus SI, Weston JH. Aspirin therapy in vernal keratoconjunctivitis. Am J Ophthalmol 1983;95:502–505.
86. Tinkelman D, Rupp G, Kaufman H, et al. Double-masked, paired-comparison clinical study of ketorolac tromethamine 0.5% ophthalmic solution compared with placebo eyedrops in the treatment of seasonal allergic conjunctivitis. Surv Ophthalmol 1993;38(suppl):133–140.
87. Buckley DC, Caldwell DR, Reaves TA. Treatment of vernal conjunctivitis with suprofen, a topical non-steroidal antiinflammatory agent. Invest Ophthalmol Vis Sci 1986;27:29–37.

88. Wood TS, Stewart RH, Bowman RW, et al. Suprofen treatment of contact lens-associated giant papillary conjunctivitis. Ophthalmology 1988;95:822–826.

89. Bishop K, Abelson MB, Cheetham J, Harper D. Evaluation of flurbiprofen in the treatment of antigen-induced allergic conjunctivitis. Invest Ophthalmol Vis Sci 1990;31(suppl):487.

90. Bleik JH, Tabbara KF. Topical cyclosporine in vernal keratoconjunctivitis. Ophthalmology 1991;98:1679–1684.

91. BenEzra D. The role of cyclosporine eyedrops in ocular inflammatory diseases. Ocular Immunol Inflamm 1993;1:159–162.

92. Holland EJ, Olsen TW, Ketcham JM, et al. Topical cyclosporin A in the treatment of anterior segment inflammatory disease. Cornea 1993;12:413–419.

93. Floyd R, Kalpaxis J, Thayer T, Rangus K. Double-blind comparison of HEPP (IgE pentapeptide) 0.5% ophthalmic solution (H) and sodium cromolyn ophthalmic solution, USP 4% (O) in patients having allergic conjunctivitis. Invest Ophthalmol Vis Sci 1988;29(suppl):45.

94. Noon L, Cantab BC. Prophylactic inoculation against hay fever. Lancet 1911;June 10:1572–1573.

95. Bousquet J, Michel FB. Advances in specific immunotherapy. Clin Exp Allergy 1992;22:889–896.

96. Nakagawa T. The role of IgG subclass antibodies in the clinical response to immunotherapy in allergic disease. Clin Exp Allergy 1991;21:289–296.

97. Gleich GJ, Jacob GL, Yuninger JW, Henderson LL. Measurement of the absolute levels of IgE antibodies in patients with ragweed hay fever: effect of immunotherapy on seasonal changes and relationship to IgG antibodies. J Allergy Clin Immunol 1977;60:188–198.

98. Durham SR, Ying S, Varney VA, et al. Grass pollen immunotherapy inhibits allergen-induced infiltration of CD4+ T lymphocytes and eosinophils in the nasal mucosa and increases the number of cells expressing messenger RNA for interferon-γ. J Allergy Clin Immunol 1996;97:1356–1365.

99. Litwin A, Flanagan M, Entis G, et al. Immunologic effects of encapsulated short ragweed extract: a potent new agent for oral immunotherapy. Ann Allergy Asthma Immunol 1996;77:132–138.

100. Gordon BR. Immunotherapy basics. Otolaryngol Head Neck Surg 1995;113:597–602.

CHAPTER 5

Local and Systemic Autoimmunity Affecting the Eye

People who have lost one eye from injury frequently become blind in the other eye.*

Autoimmunity, the immune attack of one's own cells and tissues, results from either a failure or breakdown in the mechanisms normally responsible for maintaining self-tolerance.[1] Ocular tissues may become the target of autoimmune attack directly or indirectly through mimicry with antigens on microorganisms or other tissues or both. When autoimmunity develops, it is characterized by immune cell infiltration and inflammation in the target tissue. In the eye, the term *uveitis* has been used to describe intraocular inflammation involving the uveal tract that is caused by infection or autoimmunity. It has become increasingly clear, however, that in many cases of uveitis, the uveal tract acts primarily as a conduit for the movement of cells to the real targets of immune attack: the retina and sclera.[2,3] Thus, the term *uveitis* is commonly used to describe intraocular inflammation involving not only the uvea but also the retina, vitreous, and sclera.[2] The term *uveoretinitis* is used to describe inflammation affecting the uvea and retina alone. A classification of the types of uveitis is shown in Table 5.1. Certainly, many instances of uveitis can be traced to an offending organism, including *Toxoplasma gondii*, herpes simplex

---

*A description of what was later referred to as *sympathetic ophthalmia* by Hippocrates (459–355 BC), as quoted by B. Samuel and A. Fuch in *Clinical Pathology of the Eye: A Practical Treatise of Histopathology*, 1952, p. 148, and referenced by KW To, FA Jakobiec, LE Zimmerman. In DM Albert, FA Jakobiec (eds), *Atlas of Clinical Ophthalmology*, Philadelphia: Saunders, 1996.

TABLE 5.1
Classifying Uveitis

Anatomic Position	Lesion Pattern	Clinical Course	Pathology	Laterality
Anterior	Diffuse	Acute	Granulomatous	Unilateral
Iritis	Distinct	Subacute	Nongranulo-	Bilateral
Iridocyclitis	Focal	Recurrent	matous	
Cyclitis	Multifocal	Chronic		
Intermediate	Disseminated			
Pars planitis				
Posterior				
Choroiditis				
Chorioretinitis				
Retinochoroiditis				
Retinitis				
Panuveitis				

Source: DK Roberts (ed). Ocular Disease: Diagnosis and Treatment (2nd ed). Boston: Butterworth–Heinemann, 1996;524.

virus (HSV), and fungi. Bacterial products such as endotoxin can also induce an ocular inflammatory response. In fact, an experimental form of uveitis, termed *endotoxin-induced uveitis*, can be induced in animals by the injection of endotoxin.[4]

Noninfectious or idiopathic uveitis is of unknown etiology and presumed to be mediated by autoimmune mechanisms. Like many autoimmune diseases, idiopathic uveitis tends to be associated with certain HLA haplotypes. Anterior uveitis, by far the most common type, affects the iris and ciliary body and is closely linked to major histocompatibility complex (MHC) class I antigens; posterior uveitis, affecting the posterior choroid and retina, is more frequently associated with certain MHC class II antigens. As we will see, further support for an autoimmune etiology comes from data showing direct immune-mediated reactivity to ocular antigens, including S antigen (S-Ag), found in the outer photoreceptor segments; interphotoreceptor retinol binding protein (IRBP), an extracellular protein involved in the transport of vitamin A derivatives between the retinal pigment epithelium and the photoreceptors; and melanin found in the iris and choroid. Finally, the fact that some diseases can be successfully treated with immunosuppression or specific antigen-tolerance induction also supports an autoimmune etiology.

This chapter discusses some of the more common ocular diseases stemming from direct or systemic autoimmunity. We begin with a general discussion of the signs and symptoms of idiopathic or autoimmune uveitis. A discussion follows of an animal model of autoimmune uveitis that has been instrumental in elucidating the etiopathogenesis of the human disease as well as in the development of potential therapeutic strategies. The remainder of the chapter describes ocular autoimmune diseases that result from direct autoimmune attack and those that develop secondarily in response to systemic autoimmune disease. A listing of these diseases, their HLA associations, and target antigens is shown in Table 5.2.

Signs and Symptoms of Uveitis

Uveitis is characterized by pain, photophobia, increased lacrimation, and blurred vision. Pathologic signs include ciliary injection, prostaglandin-induced pupillary miosis, and keratic precipitates (KPs), the latter of which consist of clusters of white blood cells that adhere to the corneal endothelium.[5] These cells originate in the vasculature of the iris, enter the aqueous humor, and travel by way of a convection current to the cornea. KPs are classified in many different ways; one noteworthy classification is mutton-fat KPs, which are indicative of a granulomatous type of inflammation. Iris nodules (Koeppe and Busacca) represent clumps of inflammatory cells on the surface of the iris and are more common during granulomatous inflammation.

Active inflammation of the iris and ciliary body results in the release of inflammatory cells and serum protein into the aqueous humor. The degree to which these elements have entered the aqueous humor, which is normally deficient in these components, is graded on an arbitrary scale measuring cells and flare, respectively. Synechiae, most often of the posterior type in which there is adhesion of the iris to the lens (Color Plate VI), can develop in anterior uveitis as a result of inflammation. If left untreated, the adhesions can become permanent and affect pupillary mobility as well as intraocular pressure, leading to secondary glaucoma.

Experimental Autoimmune Uveoretinitis

Much of what is known about the etiopathogenesis of autoimmune eye disease resulting in potentially sight-threatening uveitis has come from work in a rodent model. *Experimental autoimmune uveoretinitis* (EAU) can be induced in certain strains of rats and mice by the injection of either S-Ag or IRBP in complete Freund's adjuvant. Ten to 14 days after immunization, the animals develop a bilateral uveoretinitis. EAU was shown to be primarily mediated by T cells; disease could not be induced in nude rats (animals devoid of thymus-derived T cells) unless they were reconstituted with lymphocytes from normal animals.[6–8] Cell lines developed from lymph nodes that drain the site of antigen immunization[9] were shown to be CD4+, to proliferate in the presence of retinal antigens, and

TABLE 5.2
Ocular Autoimmune Diseases

Disease	HLA Association	Mimicry	Target Antigen(s)
Mooren's ulcer	—	Helminth Hepatitis C virus	Cornea-associated antigen
Sympathetic ophthalmia	Type I: A11, B40 Type II: DR4/DRw53, DR4/DQw3	*Mycoplasma?* Virus?	Retinal pigment epithelium
Reiter's disease	Type I: B27	*Shigella* *Campylobacter* *Yersinia* *Salmonella* *Chlamydia*	?
Ankylosing spondylitis	Type I: B27	*Yersinia* *Klebsiella*	?
Rheumatoid arthritis	Type II: DR1, DR4	Hepatitis B virus Newcastle virus Rubella virus Epstein-Barr virus *Mycoplasma?*	?
Behçet's disease	Type I: B51	Herpes simplex virus *Streptococcus*	Retinal antigens Heat shock protein-60
Vogt-Koyanagi-Harada	Type I: B54 Type II: DRβ1*0405, DQ4, DR53, DR4	?	S-antigen Müller cells
Sarcoidosis	Type II: DR3, DQ2, DRβ1	Retrovirus Mycobacteria	?
Cicatricial pemphigoid	Type II: DQw7	?	Kalinin Laminin-6 Beta 4-integrin BP180
Systemic lupus erythematosus	Type II: DR2, DR3	Type C retrovirus	DNA RNA Calreticulin
Primary Sjögren's syndrome	Type II: DR3, DR52, DQA, DQB	?	Ribonucleoproteins -SS-A (Ro RNA) -SS-B (La snRNP) Golgi complex α-Fodrin M3 muscarinic acetylcholine receptor in the lacrimal gland

to be capable of inducing EAU when transferred to naive hosts, confirming the dominant role of T cells in this disease.

Histochemical analysis of the cellular infiltrate induced in EAU suggests that T cells, primarily CD4+, appear early in the inflammatory response. As the condition progresses and CD4+ begins to dissipate, CD4+ T cells are supplanted by CD8+ T cells. Other cells recruited into the eye during the inflammatory phase include neutrophils and mast cells.[9] The immunosuppressive agents cyclosporin and FK506 have been found to be effective in treating severe sight-threatening uveitis and in preventing its development in animals.[10-12] These agents, as well as anti-inflammatory steroids and drugs that inhibit immune cell replication, are also used for the treatment of human uveitis. The development of EAU was delayed and its severity diminished by the treatment of recipient animals with anti-class II MHC,[13] intercellular adhesion molecule–1 (ICAM-1), and leukocyte function associated antigen–1 (LFA-1) antibodies.[14] These latter two molecules play an important role in the homing of lymphocytes (which express LFA-1) to their target organ (which expresses ICAM-1 on vascular endothelial cells). The expression of EAU was also modulated through T cell vaccination[15] and antigen feeding.[16,17] The latter approach, called *oral tolerance*, is thought to be mediated by regulatory immune cells that line the gastrointestinal mucosa and normally play a role in suppressing immunity to antigens in food. The National Eye Institute completed a phase I/II clinical trial comparing oral administration of retinal antigens with a placebo in patients with severe uveitis, with promising results.[18] The oral tolerance approach is also being investigated for the treatment of other autoimmune diseases, including type I diabetes, multiple sclerosis, and rheumatoid arthritis (RA).

Autoimmune Eye Diseases in the Absence of Systemic Involvement

Mooren's Ulcer

Clinical Features

Mooren's ulcer is an idiopathic condition in which the cornea undergoes progressive ulceration from the perilimbal area toward the central cornea. In its more severe presentation, it is bilateral and may extend peripherally toward the sclera.[19] Generally, Mooren's ulcer begins as gray patches of infiltrate that coalesce (Color Plate VII). The leading edge is generally elevated and progressively destroys the epithelium and anterior stroma, leaving a thinned, vascularized stroma in its wake.[20] In general, as the ulcer advances, stromal destruction precedes epithelial destruction. Repeated fluorescein applications can be used to follow the extent of epithelial loss.[21] Patients with Mooren's ulcer experience intense pain, as well as photophobia and increased lacrimation.[21] Additionally, patients may experience an anterior uveitis and secondary glaucoma, as well as cataract formation.[21] Clinicians have described two types of Mooren's ulcer.[22] The more common benign form occurs in older patients, is unilateral, and responds well to surgical intervention. The severe form occurs in younger people, is bilateral in about 75% of cases, is refractory to various treatment strategies, and is more progressive, often resulting in perforations.[20] Young African blacks, particularly Nigerians, are hardest hit.[21]

Etiology and Pathogenesis

Historically, Mooren's ulcer was thought to be a result of metabolic disorders, hereditary disease, neurotrophic disorders, and infectious agents.[23] Of these, infectious agents are now thought to play a role in the etiology of bilateral disease by inducing an autoimmune attack on the cornea. An immune system role is supported by the demonstration of large numbers of neutrophils, lymphocytes, and plasma cells, as well as increased numbers of mast cells and eosinophils in the cornea and adjacent conjunctiva.[24–26] Antibodies and activated complement proteins have also been reported.[27–29]

Perhaps the earliest firm association made between an infectious agent and Mooren's ulcer was in the case of the parasitic disease helminthiasis.[30,31] When treated for systemic helminthiasis, the ulcerative process was halted in the patients afflicted with this parasitic disease.[21] Corneal involvement in helminthiasis was speculated to be a result of either a worm-induced alteration in corneal antigens or a deposition of parasitic antigens in the cornea[21,32]; both of these conditions resulted in an immunologic attack on the cornea. Autoimmune attack of the cornea has also been suggested to result from mimicry involving the hepatitis C virus (HCV). Chronic HCV infection was shown to be associated with Mooren's ulcer in at least three patients,[33,34] which remitted with interferon alfa-2b (an antiviral agent) treatment. A role for autoimmune processes is also supported by the presence of autoantibodies directed against a unique cornea-associated antigen (CO-Ag) purified from stromal extracts.[35] CO-Ag appears to be a corneal calcium-binding protein.[36] The damage inflicted by these antibodies in the peripheral cornea is facilitated by the normally high concentration of the complement protein C1 found in that region. Complement activation results not only in the direct lysis of corneal cells, but also in the recruitment of damaging inflammatory cells. Other evidence for an autoimmune etiology in Mooren's ulcer includes the predisposition to the disease following ocular surgical procedures or trauma,[20] the accumulation of large numbers of CD4+ T cells and B cells in the peripheral cornea[37,38] and the aberrant expression of MHC class II antigens on corneal epithelial and stromal cells.[21,38]

Treatment

Initial treatment requires aggressive use of topical 1% prednisolone acetate twice an hour until progression of the ulcer is halted, followed by a tapering until resolution is achieved.[20] Another strategy includes the use of topical or systemic cyclosporin A immunosuppression,[39,40] which suppresses T cell help for antibody production and results in an increase in suppressor T cells. Surgical excision of the perilimbal conjunctiva to remove the source of antibodies and inflammatory cells has been effective in refractory cases.[21] Even though keratoplasty may be performed as a last resort, these patients represent a high risk for rejection or recurrence of the ulcer.[41]

Sympathetic Ophthalmia

Clinical Features

Sympathetic ophthalmia (SO) is a relatively rare ocular disorder that develops after surgical or, more often, traumatic ocular penetration.[42,43] After anywhere from 5 days to as long as nearly 7 decades after injury, a granulomatous uveitis develops in the traumatized eye, called the *exciting* eye, as well as in the initially unaffected *sympathizing* eye.[44,45] Most cases occur within 1 year of ocular penetration.[46] Patients usually present with pain, photophobia, and a decreased visual acuity in both eyes.[46] The uveitis characteristic of this syndrome is granulomatous, exhibiting mutton-fat KPs, ciliary injection, iris nodules, and posterior synechiae. One of the earliest signs may be the presence of cells in the retrolenticular region.[44] Mononuclear infiltration and thickening of the choroid, as well as vitreitis, are also seen.

Two characteristic histopathologic findings are the presence of Dalen-Fuchs nodules and lack of involvement of the choriocapillaris (Color Plate VIII). Dalen-Fuchs nodules, which are not pathognomonic for SO, consist of an aggregation of macrophages (in many cases epithelioid in nature), retinal pigment epithelial cells, and T cells internal to Bruch's membrane.[46–48] Although classically thought to involve the choroid and not the retina, many patients do show photoreceptor destruction or retinal vasculitis.[49] Optic nerve head and subretinal edema can also occur and can contribute to exudative retinal detachment.[44] Extraocular symptoms occur in a small minority of patients with SO and take the form of vitiligo, alopecia, poliosis, hearing loss, and meningeal irritation.[46,50] These are also manifested in Vogt-Koyanagi-Harada (VKH) disease. In fact, the clinical picture in both diseases is very similar except for the fact that SO does not affect the choriocapillaris and does not result in chorioretinal scarring, which are common in VKH.[51]

Etiology and Pathogenesis

Unlike the uveitis and inflammation seen in many cases of idiopathic ocular diseases, the causative factor in SO, ocular penetration, is known. It is conceivable that ocular penetration facilitates the entry of infectious agents into the eye, which could trigger the disease. Although various pathogenic organisms have been suggested as etiologic agents in SO, such as viruses and *Mycoplasma*,[52] no firm evidence supports their involvement. A more accepted view is that penetrating injury results in the release of previously immunologically sequestered ocular antigens to which the immune system had not been made tolerant, leading to an autoimmune response. These antigens gain entry into the conjunctiva or other areas that drain via lymphatic vessels into regional lymph nodes. Bacteria entering through the open wound could play an adjuvant role in stimulating antiocular immunity.[46] Parenthetically, it should be noted that it is hard to reconcile this theory with the cases of SO that occur many years after ocular trauma.

Reports of cell-mediated and humoral-immune responses to uveoretinal extracts support the theory that SO represents a trauma-induced autoimmunity to ocular antigens.[53–56] Immunization of animals with uveal extracts caused an ocular inflammatory response similar to SO.[57,58] Peripheral blood lymphocytes from patients proliferate when stimulated with retinal pigment epithelium and retinal antigen but not with choroidal extract. This latter finding supports the hypothesis that the disclosing of previously sequestered antigens (i.e., rctinal antigens) plays an important etiologic role in the disease. As in other autoimmune diseases, there is an association of SO with certain MHC haplotypes, specifically in this case with the class I types HLA-A11 and B40 and the class II types DR4/DRw53 and DR4/DQw3.[46]

Treatment

It is generally accepted that if the traumatized eye cannot be saved it should be removed immediately, or at most within 2 weeks.[59] Drug therapy involves the use of high doses of systemic and topical corticosteroids, which are gradually tapered over a 3-month period in conjunction with cycloplegic agents. The second line of therapeutic agents includes the immunosuppressive agent cyclosporin and the cytotoxic agent chlorambucil, which inhibits lymphocyte proliferation.

Autoimmune Eye Diseases with Systemic Involvement

Diseases with Joint Involvement

Reiter's Disease

Clinical Features.   Reiter's disease shares many clinical features with other seronegative spondyloarthropathies, such as ankylosing spondylitis (AKS), particularly the lack of association with rheumatoid factors or nodules, anterior segment involvement, and a strong association with MHC class I antigen HLA-B27.[60] Patients with Reiter's disease usually manifest urethritis or cervicitis early in the course of the disease, as well as arthritis and mucopurulent conjunctivitis.[61] Mucosal or cutaneous lesions, or both, may also be present. The arthritis preferentially affects the larger joints and the weight-bearing joints of the legs, particularly the sacroiliac joints. Unlike in ankylosing spondylitis, the vertebral column is less involved. Tendonitis, especially involving the muscles of the lower back as well as the Achilles' tendon, is common, with the latter being involved relatively early in the course of the disease. Reiter's disease is a recurrent disease. Acute attacks that last a few months are separated by quiescent periods.[60] Although some patients with self-limiting disease go through only a few of these cycles, a significant number have chronic relapsing disease exhibiting potentially high morbidity.[62,63]

The ocular manifestations of this disease often precede or present concurrently with arthritis or urethritis. The presenting ocular manifestation may be iridocyclitis. Other ocular manifestations include mucopurulent conjunctivitis, episcleritis, papillitis, and superficial punctate or infiltrative keratitis.[61,64] Recurrent disease is most often associated with acute iridocyclitis, accompanied by heavy cells and flare, which, in severe cases, can result in posterior synechiae.[65]

Etiology and Pathogenesis.   Reiter's disease preferentially strikes men in their 20s and 30s. It has been suggested that the incidence in women may be somewhat higher than reported because of the presence of occult cervicitis.[60] As mentioned, Reiter's disease develops most frequently in patients that express the HLA-B27 class I MHC antigen,[66] though there is less of such an association in blacks.[67] HLA-B27 presents bacterial antigen to class I restricted cytotoxic CD8+ T cells, facilitating the inflammatory response. Various bacteria, including *Shigella, Campylobacter, Yersinia, Klebsiella, Salmonella,* and *Chlamydia,* have been implicated in the development of Reiter's disease.[68] The frequency of development of reactive arthritis and uveitis after a bout with any dysenteric or sexually transmitted organisms, including human immunodeficiency virus, is quite high.

There have been reports of the isolation of infectious agents from synovial fluid and membranes, urethras, and conjunctivas in these patients.[69] When *Chlamydia,* isolated from synovial membranes, was injected into rabbit eyes, the sequelae resembled the ocular manifestations of Reiter's disease.[70] The immune response to these organisms may be inadequate because they present epitopes resembling self-epitopes to which the immune system has been made tolerant. In many cases, however, patients are seronegative at the time of disease presentation.

Treatment.   For self-limiting disease, systemic symptoms are treated with nonsteroidal anti-inflammatory drugs (NSAIDs) such as naproxen.[60] More aggressive forms may require the use of systemic immunosuppressive agents and lymphocytotoxic agents such as methotrexate and azathioprine.[71-73] Ocular disease is treated aggressively with topical corticosteroids, mydriatics, and vasoconstrictors to prevent the tissue damage associated with iridocyclitis.

Ankylosing Spondylitis

Clinical Features.   In many ways, the patient profile for AKS is similar to Reiter's syndrome. Patients tend to be men in their 20s or 30s who experience inflammatory arthritis in their sacroiliac joints and iridocyclitis. AKS is one of the more common systemic diseases associated with uveitis.[74-76] Unlike patients with Reiter's syndrome, AKS patients have preferential and significant arthritis of the spine that may become severe enough to interfere with vertebral flexion and chest expansion. About half of the patients are asymptomatic.[77] Typical arthritic symptoms include lower back pain and stiffness and pain in the sacroiliac joints.[77]

Etiology and Pathogenesis.   AKS, like Reiter's syndrome, is far more prevalent in individuals expressing the HLA-B27 haplotype. As explained above, the propensity to develop disease in these individuals likely relates to an antecedent bacterial infection. In the case of AKS, the bacteria that have been implicated are *Yersinia enterocolitica* and *Klebsiella*.[78] Molecular mimicry between HLA-B27 and the nitrogenase and pullulanase D molecules in the *Klebsiella* microbe has been reported.[79] In addition, an association exists between a polymorphism at the LMP2 locus of HLA-B27 and the development of acute anterior uveitis in AKS patients.[80]

Treatment.   The mainstay of therapy for most patients with AKS is systemic NSAIDs, including aspirin. Combination therapy of anti-CD4 and anti–IL-6 monoclonal antibodies has also been used experimentally in severe cases.[81] As in Reiter's syndrome, the ocular symptoms are treated with topical steroids and cycloplegic agents. In general, ocular treatment is aggressive to prevent the secondary complications of posterior synechiae, secondary glaucoma, and cystoid macular edema.[61]

Rheumatoid Arthritis

Clinical Features.   RA is an inflammatory joint disease classically described as an additive, asymmetric, deforming polyarthritis.[82] Patients experience morning joint stiffness and arthritis in three or more joint areas with at least one joint affected in the hand. In general, the metacarpal joints are affected early in the course of the disease, followed by involvement of the shoulder, elbow, knee, and ankle joints. X-rays reveal significant bone erosion at the joint margins, as well as ancillary damage to the

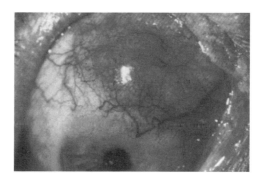

FIGURE 5.1. Nodular scleritis in rheumatoid arthritis. Note area of scleral inflammation with nodule formation as well as an area anterior to nodule showing loss of sclera from a previous inflammatory episode. (Reprinted with permission from DM Albert, FA Jakobiec [eds], Atlas of Clinical Ophthalmology. Philadelphia: Saunders, 1996;488.)

soft tissue surrounding the joints; the latter is responsible for the characteristic ulnar deviation of the fingers.[82,83] In addition to the joints, several other connective tissue regions are affected in this disease. About one-third of patients display cutaneous or subcutaneous nodules characterized by fibrinoid necrosis and inflammation.[84] Pulmonary nodules, effusions, and interstitial fibrosis are also seen.[82] Less common extra-articular features include pericarditis and anemia.

Ocular complications occur in the mid-to-later stages of the disease in about one-fourth of patients. The three most common ocular complications include secondary Sjögren's syndrome (SS), scleritis, and rheumatoid corneal melts. SS, or keratoconjunctivitis sicca, is seen in up to one-fourth of RA patients and can lead to the development of secondary bacterial keratitis. Inflammation of the sclera in the form of scleritis or episcleritis is also seen in a significant minority of patients. Episcleritis tends to be self-limiting and is less frequently associated with severe ocular complications and systemic disease.[82] Scleritis can be severe, however, and could lead to scleromalacia perforans, ectasia formation, and perforation of the globe (Figure 5.1).[85] Scleritis generally precedes or parallels the onset of systemic symptoms,[86] which tend to be more severe and occur with a greater frequency of extra-articular manifestations[82,87] than in patients not exhibiting scleritis. Patients with necrotizing scleritis tend to have a worse prognosis in part because of the development of vasculitis.[88] Retinal vasculitis was reported to occur in about 18% of RA patients.[89] Noninflammatory or necrotizing marginal corneal ulcers, called *rheumatoid corneal melts*, are also seen in RA patients.[82] The ocular manifestations of the juvenile form of RA are acute and chronic iridocyclitis.[90]

Etiology and Pathogenesis.   RA strikes about 2% of the population, with women affected about three times more frequently than men.[82] Most patients have circulating autoantibodies in their blood, called *rheumatoid factor* (RF), that are directed against their own IgG molecules. Autoantibody production may be induced by an alteration in the structure of targeted IgG molecules.[91] Other targets for autoantibodies include double-stranded DNA[92] and collagen.[93] It is important to note that the presence of RF is neither necessary nor sufficient for the diagnosis of RA.[82] The role of RF and the humoral immune system in general in the pathogenesis of RA is unknown. These antibodies form circulating immune complexes, which may deposit along vessel walls and contribute to the development of vasculitis in a small number of cases.

Although the synovium in RA patients is replete with B cells and RF-secreting plasma cells, it also contains constituents of the cellular arm of immunity, in particular, polymorphonuclear leukocytes and T cells. A role for cellular immune mechanisms in RA is further suggested by the in vitro demonstration of T cell reactivity to synovial and ocular antigens by macrophages,[94] as well as T cell cytotoxicity directed against synovial cells.[95] Although there have been reports of depressed cellular immunity to non–disease-related antigens, subset analysis failed to reveal any consistent abnormalities in the numbers or percentages of either CD4+ or CD8+ cells.[82]

RA is associated with the HLA class II types DR4 and DR1. More than 90% of patients with RA have one or the other or both of these haplotypes.[96] These haplotypes may be particularly well suited to present antigens that trigger the disease; what this antigen is remains to be elucidated. As with other joint and ocular diseases, mimicry with antigens present on microorganisms and viruses has been suggested, including hepatitis B, Newcastle, rubella, and Epstein-Barr viruses.[97,98] The attempts at isolating *Mycoplasma* organisms from the joints of RA patients have been inconclusive,[97] though long-term RA patients produce *Mycoplasma* antibodies.[99] An association has also been suggested between RA patients expressing ocular complications and certain cytokine genes such as those that encode IL-1.[100]

Treatment.   Initial treatment of RA involves the use of NSAIDs, such as aspirin, naproxen, and indomethacin. The antimalarial drug hydroxychloroquine is used in more severe cases to induce remission,[101] but its dosage is limited because of its ocular toxicity.[102] Specifically, hydroxychloroquine accumulates in the retinal pigment epithelium and may produce a pigmentary retinopathy. The most widely used drug is methotrexate, which has been found to be efficacious, though long-term treatment is required. Severe forms of the disease can also be treated with immunosuppressive agents such as cyclophosphamide and azathioprine. Topical steroids are used to treat episcleritis, but systemic steroids are generally required to treat scleritis. Slow-release artificial tear inserts are effective in the treatment of dry eye in RA patients.[103]

Two relatively new treatment modalities for inflammatory joint disease are oral tolerance and the use of anticytokine antibodies. As mentioned earlier, oral tolerance involves the ingestion of a specific target antigen, resulting in a downregulation of immune responsiveness to the antigen in much the same way that immune reactivity to the abundant antigens in our food is suppressed. The antigen used to suppress RA is collagen type II.[104] The use of anti tumor necrosis factor (anti-TNF) monoclonal antibodies has also been effective and supports a leading role for this cytokine in the orchestration of joint inflammation.[105] Both of these types of intervention are referred to as *immunotherapy.*

Behçet's Disease

Clinical Features.   Behçet's disease is a multisystem disorder characterized by recurrent episodes of aphthous ulcerations of the mouth and genitalia and uveitis.[106] Patients may also demonstrate arthritis in the knees, intestinal ulcers, epididymitis, vascular disease, meningomyelitis, and neuropsychiatric symptoms.[107] Ocular manifestations occur in 75% of patients and take the form of a nongranulomatous uveitis[108] that develops about 2–3 years after the initial symptoms appear.[109] Most cases take the form of iridocyclitis, many with an accompanying hypopyon that may only be visible with a slit lamp. Recurrent anterior segment inflammation can lead to angle-closure glaucoma.[107] Of the most concern is the propensity of some patients to develop retinal vasoocclusive episodes that irreversibly damage the retina.[107] Retinal vasculitis and retinitis result in diffuse serous, exudative, and hemorrhagic leakage throughout the fundus, as well as optic disc edema and atrophy.[106] Other ocular symptoms include conjunctivitis, scleritis, and keratitis.

Etiology and Pathogenesis.   Behçet's disease is most prevalent in men living in the Middle and Far East and men descended from such populations. The highest incidence of disease in the United States is in the state of Minnesota, where the incidence is 1 in 300,000. The disease is most associated with the class I MHC haplotype HLA-B51, though the HLA-B51 gene itself may not be the pathogenic gene but rather an as yet unidentified gene closely linked to it.[110] Immunopathologic studies have implicated autoreactive antibodies, neutrophils, and lymphocytes in disease pathogenesis. Although there is evidence that immune complexes play a role in the perivasculitis associated with this disease,[111,112] only about one-third of patients were found to have such complexes; furthermore, their presence was associated with quiescent periods of disease.[113]

Various cell types that mediate the cellular arm of immunity have been implicated in Behçet's disease. Neutrophil hyperfunction has been suggested as an etiologic factor, and mast cells were shown to play a role in the development of skin ulcerations. T cells seem to play a particularly important role, as they are present in skin lesions and ocular inflammation.[114,115] Patients display a reduced CD4/CD8 ratio[116] and have elevated serum levels of IL-2 and interferon gamma (IFN-γ).[117,118] Specifically in the eye, the retinal perivascular infiltrate was shown to comprise activated CD4+ T cells,[119] and patients demonstrated a specific T cell response to retinal antigens.[120] T cell reactivity was also demonstrated to heat shock protein (HSP)-60, which resembles, in part, the HSP-65 molecule of mycobacteria, *Streptococcus sanguis*, and HSV, suggesting a role for mimicry in the etiology of the disease.[121,122]

Treatment.   The ocular symptoms of Behçet's disease are usually more severe than the other systemic manifestations. Patients with mild iridocyclitis may be treated with topical steroids, but most patients require systemic steroids at presentation. Other drugs that are used following an initial regimen of steroids include the immunosuppressants cyclosporin and FK506 and colchicine, which is thought to suppress leukocyte migration and phagocytosis. The theory that viruses such as HSV may be important in disease etiology is supported by the successful long-term treatment of a patient with IFN-α and -γ.[123]

Systemic Lupus Erythematosus

Clinical Features.   Systemic lupus erythematosus (SLE) is a multisystem autoimmune disorder associated with the HLA-DR2 and -DR3 class II haplotypes. Many more women than men develop the disease, and black women are particularly affected. To establish a diagnosis of SLE, a minimum of four criteria out of a list of 11 must be met. Some of the more common findings are a malar rash, arthritis, oral ulcers, renal disorders, and central nervous system involvement such as seizures, organic brain syndrome, or psychosis.[124] Nearly all patients experience fatigue, low-grade fever, and weight loss,[125,126] most commonly at presentation. The diagnosis is also made on an immunologic basis, particularly by the demonstration of antinuclear antibodies.

A host of ocular tissues are affected in up to almost one-third of patients with SLE,[127] many as a result of focal vasculitis, though severe visual loss is uncommon. Marginal telangiectasia and erythematous patches are common on the eyelids and up to 20% of patients develop non-specific conjunctivitis and keratitis.[128] Secondary SS and neuro-ophthalmic lesions are also seen, the latter of which can take the form of cranial nerve palsy, retrobulbar optic neuritis, nystagmus, diplopia, brain stem ophthalmoplegias, and pseudotumors.[128–130] Retinal involvement usually takes the form of cotton-wool spots at the sites of retinal infarcts and superficial hemorrhages (Color Plate IX). A small number of patients can develop severe retinal vasoocclusive disease with associated poor visual outcome.[131]

Etiology and Pathogenesis.   SLE is thought to represent a classic case of a type III hypersensitivity disease resulting from the deposition of circulating and in situ immune complexes. Immunopathogenic analyses revealed B cell hyperactivity in these patients, exemplified by polyclonal B cell activation, hypergammaglobulinemia, and autoantibody formation. B cell receptor–initiated events were found to be increased in SLE and patient T cells were shown to express increased CD40 ligand, a molecule necessary for T cells to provide help to B cells for the production of T dependent antigens.[132] A functional deficiency in a subset of CD4+ helper T cells that induces the activation of suppressor CD8+ T cells has also been suggested. The development of anti-DNA antibodies is a hallmark of SLE.[133] Other target antigens for autoantibodies in SLE patients include RNA; calreticulin, an intracellular calcium-binding protein found in the cytoplasm and nucleus[134,135]; and type C human endogenous retroviral particles.[136]

Why these patients develop autoantibodies is unknown, but mimicry has been suggested in light of the demonstration of antibodies to type C viral particles and their identification on the lymphocytes and in the kidneys and lungs of some patients.[137,138] Viruses have also been implicated in the development of the animal form of SLE which develops in New Zealand black mice. It was speculated that these viral particles may be transmitted genetically and as a result would be recognized as "self" by the immune system, allowing them to attack regulatory immune cells with impunity and leading to an imbalance which results in autoantibody formation. As a final note, as in cicatricial pemphigoid (CP), SLE can be induced by drugs, particularly procainamide, quinidine, isoniazid, sulfasalazine, and acebutolol.[139]

Treatment. For the less severe effects of SLE such as arthritis, NSAIDs, such as indomethacin, low-dose prednisolone, and hydroxychloroquine, have been used, though the latter can cause retinal damage. The more serious complications are controlled by systemic steroids. Patients that do not respond well to systemic steroids are given the immunosuppressive agents cyclophosphamide and methotrexate. Plasma exchanges were reported to successfully heal one severe case of SLE with bilateral serous retinal detachment.[140]

Sjögren's Syndrome

Clinical Features. SS is an autoimmune disorder characterized by dryness of the eyes, mouth, and other mucous membranes, and it is often associated with other connective tissue diseases. When dry eyes (xerophthalmia) and mouth (xerostomia) are present alone, the disease is referred to as *primary* SS; when they are associated with other connective tissue diseases such as RA, scleroderma, or SLE, the disease is referred to as *secondary* SS.[141] As discussed below, differences in the classification of SS in the United States and abroad have contributed to ambiguities regarding the etiology of this disease.

Patients display organ-directed autoimmunity that affects exocrine gland function throughout the body. Systemic manifestations of SS include gastrointestinal mucosal atrophy, hepatobiliary disease, and pancreatitis. There is also an increased risk for the development of lymphomas. In the oral cavity, dry mouth results from salivary gland involvement. Bilateral parotid gland enlargement is seen in about half of patients,[142] with most complaining of difficulty chewing and swallowing food. Inherent dryness of the oral and nasal mucosae contributes to this finding and also results in hoarseness and epistaxis (nosebleeds).

The disease affects the lacrimal gland, resulting in the development of keratoconjunctivitis sicca, found in about 90% of patients.[143] As expected, tear breakup time is rapid and constituents of the aqueous tear film are markedly reduced. Initially, a noninfectious ropy discharge and papillary response of the conjunctiva develops as a result of chronic irritation.[142] In the initial stages of the disease, patients complain of foreign body sensation, photophobia, redness, burning, and itching. Although these patients have reduced tear production, many still exhibit a reflex tearing response. Corneal pathology may occur in severe cases as a direct result of corneal irritation or secondarily in response to bacterial infection, and, in rare cases, perforation can occur. Staphylococcal infection of the anterior surface of the eye occurs in about 75% of all cases of keratoconjunctivitis sicca.[142]

Etiology and Pathogenesis.   SS primarily afflicts women between 40 and 60 years of age. It is estimated that as many as 3% of women over 55 are affected.[144] The disease is linked to class II MHC antigens DR3, DR52, DQA, and DQB. When discussing the etiopathogenesis of primary, autoimmune SS, it is important to distinguish it from drug side effects or disease caused by HCV, Epstein-Barr virus, retroviral infection, lymphoma, autonomic neuropathy, depression, and primary fibromyalgia.[145] Hypergammaglobulinemia is a frequent finding in SS and is usually of the polyclonal type,[142] though overall T cell activity has been reported to be reduced. Primary autoimmune SS is characterized by the systemic production of autoantibodies to the ribonucleoprotein (RNP) particles SS-A, also called *Ro RNA particles*, and SS-B, also called *La snRNP*.[146] These antibodies are thought to contribute directly to the pathology seen in the disease.[147,148] A mutation in the genes encoding the transporters associated with antigen processing may be involved in this autoantibody production and could be a genetic factor that determines susceptibility.[149] Other reported targets for autoantibodies in SS include a Golgi complex autoantigen,[150] the cortical cytoskeletal protein alpha-fodrin,[146] and lacrimal gland M_3 muscarinic acetylcholine receptors.[151] SS-B autoantibodies react with fetal laminin and fetal cardiac cells, the latter of which could explain the occurrence of congenital heart block in children of mothers with these antibodies.[152]

In addition to autoantibody formation, the target organs in SS are characterized by a lymphocytic infiltrate comprising both T cells and B cells, in spite of a generalized reduction in the activity of cellular immune effectors. Evidence suggests that the activation of the target epithelial cells may play a role in the activation of T cells. This is supported by the demonstration of markedly enhanced release of IL-1α, IL-6, and TNF-α from salivary gland epithelial cells.[153] It has been reported that apoptosis is blocked in infiltrating lymphocytes but enhanced in peripheral T cells and acinar cells in SS.[154] These data provide a mechanism to account for the findings of enhanced T cellular immunity in target organs but depressed cellular immunity systemically in these patients. It also suggests that apoptosis may play an important role in acinar cell death.

Our understanding of the etiology and pathogenetic mechanisms involved in SS has been facilitated by the investigation of three animal models. The MRL/lpr mouse fails to express Fas and develops lymphoproliferative and autoimmune diseases, one of which resembles SS.[155] The nonobese diabetic (NOD) mouse spontaneously develops autoimmune type I diabetes as well as a SS-like disease.[156] The NFS/sld mouse bears an autosomal recessive mutation, resulting in sublingual gland arrest. When thymectomized 3 days after birth, the NFS/sld mouse develops significant inflammatory changes in both the salivary and lacrimal glands, implicating the thymus in the development of autoimmunity in this model.[157]

Finally, the bioavailability of androgens is thought to play a role in the development of SS. According to this theory, the breakdown of target acinar cells occurs when androgen levels fall below a critical level,[158,159] ultimately resulting in the release of tissue antigens and the development of a lymphocytic infiltrate with concomitant autoantigenic stimulation.

Treatment.   Treatment of SS is palliative in nature. Use of a room humidifier is helpful. For ocular symptoms, frequent use of artificial tears containing methylcellulose or polyvinyl alcohol may be effective, as well as the use of moisture shields at night. Insertion of nasolacrimal plugs can be used if tear replacement is insufficient.

The importance of T cells in SS was confirmed by the improvement seen in patients who were treated with systemic cyclophosphamide for the treatment of symptoms unrelated to SS. This was further supported by the findings in the MRL/lpr mouse in which successful transfer of the disease was prevented by anti-CD4 and anti–T cell receptor antibody treatment.[160] Two new treatments under investigation that have shown promising preliminary results include the use of botulinum toxin[161] and the antiviral agent IFN-α2,[162] both of which increased tearing in SS patients.

Autoimmune Eye Disease with Multisystem Involvement without Arthritis

Vogt-Koyanagi-Harada Syndrome

Clinical Features.   VKH syndrome is a bilateral, diffuse granulomatous uveitis associated with poliosis, vitiligo, alopecia, and central nervous system and auditory signs. Recall that these extraocular symptoms are also

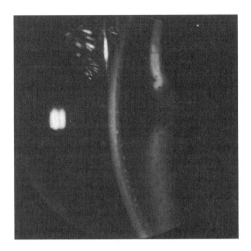

FIGURE 5.2.   Vogt-Koyanagi-Harada disease. Note granulomatous, mutton-fat keratic precipitates on the corneal endothelium. (Reprinted with permission from DM Albert, FA Jakobiec [eds], Atlas of Clinical Ophthalmology. Philadelphia: Saunders, 1996;117.)

seen in SO. The disease is more common in Asians, especially the Japanese, in whom it is responsible for about 10% of all cases of uveitis.[163,164] The extraocular findings in VKH are important in making the diagnosis. Often the disease presents as headache, nausea, vomiting, and neck stiffness, stemming from an underlying encephalopathy. Cerebrospinal fluid (CSF) analysis reveals that central nervous system inflammation is primarily a result of the infiltration by lymphocytes and monocytes.[165] Auditory signs, which often develop in conjunction with ocular symptoms, include hearing loss (higher frequencies), vertigo, and tinnitus.

Ocular disease occurs in most VKH patients and takes the form of a non-necrotizing diffuse granulomatous uveitis with mutton-fat KPs and initial sparing and late involvement of the choriocapillaris and formation of Dalen-Fuchs nodules (Figure 5.2).[164] Swelling of the ciliary body with anterior rotation and supraciliary space can cause transient angle-closure glaucoma in these patients.[166] Loss of perilimbal pigment (perilimbal vitiligo or Sugiura's sign) is seen in the great majority of Asian patients.[163,165] The most devastating ocular symptoms affect the posterior pole where inflammation leads to exudative retinal detachment and macular edema, vitreous inflammation, and optic nerve edema and hyperemia. Pigment epithelial changes with pigment migration leads to retinal depigmentation, resulting in what has been termed a *sunset glow* fundus.[167] Subretinal neovascular membranes occur in about 10% of patients and are an important cause of late vision loss.[164]

Etiology and Pathogenesis.   VKH, like many of the other diseases discussed in this chapter, has been linked to the MHC, specifically to the type

I antigen HLA-B54 and the type II antigens DR4, DRβ1*0405, DQ4, and DR53.[168] An etiologic organism was suggested by the demonstration of disease transmissibility by injection of vitreous or CSF from patients into animals,[169,170] but no agent has yet been isolated. Much evidence supports a role for autoimmune processes in this disease. Patients were shown to have an overall increase in their CD4/CD8 ratio[171] and an elevation in circulating activated cells, as determined by their expression of class II antigens.[172] In light of the clinical signs of depigmentation in various areas, it was speculated that melanin pigment was the target of autoimmune attack. Autoantibodies to uveal pigment have been described in these patients. Cell-mediated immunoreactivity has also been reported. Immune cells showed both macrophage reactivity[173] and specific cytotoxicity to melanocyte antigens.[174,175] Furthermore, melanin-laden macrophages were found in the CSF.[176]

Cellular and humoral immunity to retinal antigens has also been demonstrated. In particular, cell-mediated reactivity to S-Ag and humoral immunity to the Müller cells and the outer segments of the photoreceptors were demonstrated.[53,177] The production of IL-6 by lymphocytes in the aqueous humor was reported to play an important role as an inflammatory mediator in VKH.[178] The majority of CD4+ T cells derived from the aqueous humor of uveitic eyes expressed the memory marker CD45RO+, as well as the apoptosis-triggering antigen, Fas. Interestingly, high levels of serum IgD were found in patients with retinal vasculitis, the significance of which may relate to an abnormal state of B cell activation.[179]

Treatment.   Systemic steroid administration is the treatment of choice for VKH and, when started early, can limit disease progression. Both cyclosporin and FK506 have also been shown to be effective,[180,181] though the latter was associated with adverse side effects. Retinal detachment must be repaired quickly; laser therapy is used to repair neovascular retinal lesions.

Sarcoidosis

Clinical Features.   Sarcoidosis is an idiopathic systemic disorder characterized by the development of noncaseating granulomatous tissue.[182] Nearly all patients have respiratory involvement that takes the form of interstitial lung disease involving the alveoli, blood vessels, and bronchioles.[183] Intrathoracic and peripheral lymphadenopathy are also common, as are granulomatous involvement of the liver. A smaller number of patients develop erythema nodosum and other skin manifestations, and still fewer patients develop cardiac sarcoidosis. Many patients are asymptomatic at the time of diagnosis, which may be made based on the results of a routine chest x-ray.

Approximately 25% of patients with sarcoidosis, and in some reports up to 50%,[184] develop ocular lesions that can, in their most severe form, result in blindness. Although anterior uveitis is the most common problem, any region of the globe or ocular adnexa may be involved, including the conjunctiva, sclera, eyelids, and lacrimal gland (Color Plate X).[185] Sarcoidosis patients tend to have elevated levels of angiotensin-converting enzyme, produced by the giant cells in the granuloma, in their tears. Mutton-fat KPs are a common finding, whereas Koeppe and Busacca iris nodules develop in only about 10% of patients.[186] Patients with recurrent inflammation have an increased likelihood of developing anterior or posterior synechiae, or both, and secondary glaucoma. Other anterior segment findings are cataracts and corneal band keratopathy. Although posterior segment involvement is less common, a significant minority of patients experience inflammation of the vitreous, retina, and choroid.[187] About one-third of patients develop Dalen-Fuchs nodules.[188] Small exudates near retinal veins, termed *candle wax drippings*, may be present, but they are not a frequent finding, though many patients experience perivenous sheathing.[184,186] Decreased visual acuity may result from chronic cystoid macular edema.[184]

Etiology and Pathogenesis.   Sarcoidosis has a worldwide distribution though it has a predilection for young adults, blacks in the United States, and Scandinavians. Disease in a subgroup of patients has been linked to the class II haplotypes DR3, DQ2, as well as DRβ1.[189,190] Association of the granulomatous inflammation that occurs in this disease with mycobacterial infections has led investigators to suspect a pathogenic organism as the etiologic agent. Evidence to support this includes the demonstration of disease transmission by cardiac and bone marrow transplantation,[191,192] and the detection, by the polymerase chain reaction technique, of mycobacterial DNA in half of the patients with biopsy-proven disease.[193] Retroviruses have also been implicated in the development of sarcoidosis.[194]

It is clear from the histopathology that sarcoidosis is an immunologically mediated disease. Macrophages, the key cellular component in the granulomatous lesion, aggregate and differentiate into epithelioid and multinucleated giant cells. T and B cells as well as mast cells are also associated with the granulomatous lesion.[183] It is thought that the T cells play a role in promoting macrophage function through the release of cytokines such as IFN-γ. The proinflammatory mediators TNF-α, IL-6, and IL-1β have also been implicated.[195] Serum IgG levels and immune complexes are elevated in the serum of patients, the latter of which may contribute in small measure to the development of clinical symptoms. The role of T cells is further confirmed by the development of sarcoid granulomas in patients injected with a suspension of splenic tissue obtained from a patient with confirmed disease. Called the *Kveim test*, it is not approved by the U.S. Food and Drug Administration and is not performed in the United States for fear of infectious transmission.

Although localized granulomatous T cell activity is elevated, there have been numerous reports of depressed systemic T cell activity in these patients. Specifically, lymphocytes were shown to respond poorly to mitogens,[196] and there was reduced delayed-type hypersensitivity responsiveness to mumps and various intradermal antigens such as *Candida, Trichophyton* (a pathogenic fungus), and streptokinase-streptodornase.[197] Lymphocyte responsiveness was shown to improve in patients experiencing remission.[196]

Treatment.   The primary treatment for sarcoidosis is systemic steroids. Methotrexate, chlorambucil, and cyclosporin are also effective. Ocular sarcoidosis can be treated with topical, periocular, or systemic corticosteroids, and cycloplegia and mydriasis are sometimes necessary to prevent synechiae formation.[196]

Cicatricial Pemphigoid

Clinical Features.   CP is a blistering autoimmune disease of the mucous membranes and, less often, the skin.[198] Most patients have both oral and ocular lesions, unlike in pemphigus vulgaris, in which serious ocular involvement does not occur. Ocular involvement in CP is characterized by progressive conjunctival shrinkage, symblepharon, entropion with trichiasis, dry eye, and reduced vision from corneal opacification.[199] CP is generally staged based on the degree of conjunctival fornix shortening.[200] Patients in the initial stage experience chronic conjunctivitis with mild epitheliopathy that may affect the cornea, as well as the beginnings of subepithelial fibrosis of the conjunctiva.[201] In its final stage, patients demonstrate dry eye with ankyloblepharon and keratinization of the cornea. Although it was once thought that CP represented a dry eye syndrome that resulted from a deficiency in mucin production, this is no longer accepted. In the early stages, mucin production is normal; it is only in the later stages that goblet cell number decreases as a result of the cicatrizing process and deformation of the lids.[201] Patients with CP are at an increased risk for developing microbial colonization of the lids, lashes, conjunctiva, and cornea, and for developing microbial keratitis.

Etiology and Pathogenesis.   Most patients with CP present at a mean age of between 60 and 70 years, and there is a slight preponderance of women over men who develop the disease.[202,203] Evidence suggests that CP develops as a consequence of the development of autoantibodies, specifically of the IgG and IgA isotypes, directed against self-antigens in the epithelial basement membrane zone in the skin and eye.[204] Antigenic targets of these autoantibodies have been reported to include the proteins laminin-5 (kalinin), laminin-6,[205,206] a 168-kd protein,[207] β_4 integrin,[208] and BP180,[209,210] a hemidesmosomal glycoprotein associated with two other autoimmune blistering diseases: bullous pemphigoid and herpes gestationis.

Antibody binding to conjunctival basement membrane proteins is thought to result in complement activation, resulting in the release of mast cell mediators and the recruitment of macrophages and lymphocytes, primarily helper T cells, into the area.[201] Cytokines and other mediators released from these cells induce fibroblasts to secrete types IV and VII collagen, resulting in cicatrization. Immunochemical studies suggest that complement may not play as dominant a role as once thought.[205] Systemic immune changes indicative of autoreactive disease, such as an increase in circulating soluble IL-2 receptors, CD8 glycoprotein, and TNF-α are also seen in CP.[201] Furthermore, the development of CP is associated with the class II HLA-DQw7 gene.[211]

Some cases of conjunctival scarring are known to be drug-induced. Topical agents that have been associated with conjunctival scarring include pilocarpine, idoxuridine, epinephrine, timolol, and echothiophate iodide.[201,212] These agents produce the full range of disease symptomatology from a condition indistinguishable from CP to a more self-limiting toxic form,[199] and their mechanism of action may be equally diverse.

Treatment. The sulfa drug dapsone was shown to be effective in many cases of CP,[213] but is contraindicated in patients with glucose-6-phosphate dehydrogenase deficiency. In unresponsive cases, either azathioprine, methotrexate, or cyclophosphamide is used. In spite of the presence of large numbers of helper T cells in the CP lesion, cyclosporin has been shown to be ineffective in treating the disease.

References

1. Abbas AK, Lichtman AH, Pober JS. Cellular and Molecular Immunology. Philadelphia: Saunders, 1997;413.
2. Whitcup SM, Nussenblatt RB. Immunologic mechanisms of uveitis. New targets for immunomodulation. Arch Ophthalmol 1997;115:520–525.
3. Forrester JV, Liversidge J, Dick A, et al. What determines the site of inflammation in uveitis and chorioretinitis? Eye 1997;11:162–166.
4. Abel GS. Uveitis. In DK Roberts, JE Terry (eds), Ocular Disease: Diagnosis and Treatment. Boston: Butterworth–Heinemann, 1996;519.
5. Rosenbaum JT, McDevitt HO, Guss RB, Egbert PR. Endotoxin-induced uveitis in rats as a model for human disease. Nature 1980;286:611–613.
6. Salinas-Carmona MC, Nussenblatt RB, Gery I. Experimental autoimmune uveitis in the athymic nude rat. Eur J Immunol 1982;12:480–484.
7. Caspi RR, Chan CC, Fujino Y, et al. Recruitment of antigen-nonspecific cells plays a pivotal role in the pathogenesis of a T cell–mediated organ-specific autoimmune disease, experimental autoimmune uveoretinitis. J Neuroimmunol 1993;47:177–188.
8. Caspi RR. Experimental Autoimmune Uveoretinitis—Rat and Mouse. In IR Cohen, A Miller (eds), Autoimmune Disease Models: A Guidebook. San Diego: Academic, 1994;60.

9. Caspi RR, Roberge FG, McAllister CG, et al. T cell lines mediating experimental autoimmune uveoretinitis (EAU) in the rat. J Immunol 1986;136:928–933.

10. BenEzra D, Maftzir G, de Courten C, Timonen P. Ocular penetration of cyclosporin A. III: the human eye. Br J Ophthalmol 1990;74:350–352.

11. Kawashima H, Fujino Y, Mochizuki M. Antigen-specific suppressor cells induced by FK506 in experimental autoimmune uveoretinitis in the rat. Invest Ophthalmol Vis Sci 1990;31:2500–2507.

12. Fujino Y, Mochizuki M, Chan CC, et al. FK506 treatment of S-antigen induced uveitis in primates. Curr Eye Res 1991;10:679–690.

13. Wetzig R, Hooks JJ, Percopo CM, et al. Anti-Ia antibody diminishes ocular inflammation in experimental autoimmune uveitis. Curr Eye Res 1988;7: 809–818.

14. Whitcup SM, DeBarge LR, Caspi RR, et al. Monoclonal antibodies against ICAM-1 (CD54) and LFA-1 (CD11a/CD18) inhibit experimental autoimmune uveitis. Clin Immunol Immunopathol 1993;67:143–150.

15. Beraud E, Kotake S, Caspi RR, et al. Control of experimental autoimmune uveoretinitis by low dose T cell vaccination. Cell Immunol 1992;140:112–122.

16. Gregerson DS, Obritsch WF, Donoso LA. Oral tolerance in experimental autoimmune uveoretinitis. Distinct mechanisms of resistance are induced by low dose vs. high dose feeding protocols. J Immunol 1993;151:5751–5761.

17. Thurau SR, Chan CC, Nussenblatt RB, Caspi RR. Oral tolerance in a murine model of relapsing experimental autoimmune uveoretinitis (EAU): induction of protective tolerance in primed animals. Clin Exp Immunol 1997;109:370–376.

18. Nussenblatt RB, Gery I, Weiner HL, et al. Treatment of uveitis by oral administration of retinal antigens: results of a phase I/II randomized masked trial. Am J Ophthalmol 1997;123:583–592.

19. Spencer WH. Cornea. In WH Spencer (ed), Ophthalmic Pathology. An Atlas and Textbook. Philadelphia: Saunders, 1985;229–388.

20. Oliver GE. Diseases of the Conjunctiva, Cornea, and Sclera. In DK Roberts, JE Terry (eds), Ocular Disease: Diagnosis and Treatment. Boston: Butterworth–Heinemann, 1996;479–518.

21. Robin SB, Robin JB. Mooren's Ulcer. In JS Pepose, GN Holland, KR Wilhelmus (eds), Ocular Infection & Immunity. St. Louis: Mosby, 1996;471–473.

22. Wood TO, Kaufman HE. Mooren's ulcer. Am J Ophthalmol 1971;71(suppl): 417–422.

23. Friedlaender MH. Allergy and Immunology of the Eye (2nd ed). New York: Raven Press, 1992;196.

24. Edwards WC, Reed RE. Mooren's ulcer. A pathologic case report. Arch Ophthalmol 1968;80:361–364.

25. Mondino BJ, Brown SI, Rabin BS. Cellular immunity in Mooren's ulcer. Am J Ophthalmol 1978;85:788–791.

26. Young RD, Watson PG. Light and electron microscopy of corneal melting syndrome (Mooren's ulcer). Br J Ophthalmol 1982;66:341–356.

27. Eiferman RA, Hyndiuk R. IgE in limbal conjunctiva in Mooren's ulcer. Can J Ophthalmol 1977;12:234–236.

28. Eiferman RA, Hyndiuk RA, Hensley GT. Limbal immunopathology of Mooren's ulcer. Ann Ophthalmol 1978;10:1203–1206.

29. Foster CS, Kenyon KR, Greiner J, et al. The immunopathology of Mooren's ulcer. Am J Ophthalmol 1979;88:149–159.

30. Kietzman B. Mooren's ulcer in Nigeria. Am J Ophthalmol 1968;65:679–685.

31. Majekodunmi AA. Ecology of Mooren's ulcer in Nigeria. Doc Ophthalmol 1980;49:211–219.

32. van der Gaag R, Abdillahi H, Stilma JS, Vetter JC. Circulating antibodies against corneal epithelium and hookworm in patients with Mooren's ulcer from Sierra Leone. Br J Ophthalmol 1983;67:623–628.

33. Wilson SE, Lee WM, Murakami C, et al. Mooren-type hepatitis C virus-associated corneal ulceration. Ophthalmology 1994;101:736–745.

34. Moazami G, Auran JD, Florakis GJ, et al. Interferon treatment of Mooren's ulcers associated with hepatitis C. Am J Ophthalmol 1995;119:365–366.

35. Gottsch JD, Liu SH, Minkovitz JB, et al. Autoimmunity to a cornea-associated stromal antigen in patients with Mooren's ulcer. Invest Ophthalmol Vis Sci 1995;36:1541–1547.

36. Liu SH, Gottsch JD. Amino acid sequence of an immunogenic corneal stromal protein. Invest Ophthalmol Vis Sci 1996;37:944–948.

37. Murray PI, Rahi AH. Pathogenesis of Mooren's ulcer: some new concepts. Br J Ophthalmol 1984;68:182–187.

38. Lopez JS, Price FW Jr, Whitcup SM, et al. Immunohistochemistry of Terrien's and Mooren's corneal degeneration. Arch Ophthalmol 1991;109:988–992.

39. Zhao JC, Jin XY. Immunological analysis and treatment of Mooren's ulcer with cyclosporin A applied topically. Cornea 1993;12:481–488.

40. Wakefield D, Robinson LP. Cyclosporin therapy in Mooren's ulcer. Br J Ophthalmol 1987;71:415–417.

41. McDonnell PJ. Recurrence of Mooren's ulcer after lamellar keratoplasty. Cornea 1989;8:191–194.

42. Nussenblatt RB, Whitcup SM, Palestine AG. Uveitis. Fundamentals and Clinical Practice (2nd ed). St. Louis: Mosby, 1996;300.

43. Nussenblatt RB, Tabbara KF. Autoimmune Diseases. In KF Tabbara, RB Nussenblatt (eds), Posterior Uveitis: Diagnosis and Management. Boston: Butterworth–Heinemann, 1994;94.

44. Abel GS. Uveitis. In DK Roberts, JE Terry (eds), Ocular Disease: Diagnosis and Treatment. Boston: Butterworth–Heinemann, 1996;544.

45. Zaharia MA, Lamarche J, Laurin M. Sympathetic uveitis 66 years after injury. Can J Ophthalmol 1984;19:240–243.

46. Chan C-C, Roberge FG. Sympathetic Ophthalmia. In JS Pepose, GN Holland, KR Wilhelmus (eds), Ocular Infection and Immunity. St. Louis: Mosby, 1996;723–733.

47. Chan CC, BenEzra D, Hsu SM, et al. Granulomas in sympathetic ophthalmia and sarcoidosis. Immunohistochemical study. Arch Ophthalmol 1985;103:198–202.

48. Jakobiec FA, Marboe CC, Knowles DM 2nd, et al. Human sympathetic ophthalmia. An analysis of the inflammatory infiltrate by hybridoma-monoclonal

antibodies, immunochemistry, and correlative electron microscopy. Ophthalmology 1983;90:76–95.

49. Croxatto JO, Rao NA, McLean IW, Marak GE. Atypical histopathologic features in sympathetic ophthalmia. A study of a hundred cases. Int Ophthalmol 1982;3:129–135.

50. Goto H, Rao NA. Sympathetic ophthalmia and Vogt-Koyanagi-Harada syndrome. Int Ophthalmol Clin 1990;30:279–285.

51. Nussenblatt RB, Whitcup SM, Palestine AG. Uveitis. Fundamentals and Clinical Practice (2nd ed). St. Louis: Mosby, 1996;304.

52. Schreck E. [Further investigations for the demonstration of a specific microorganism in sympathetic ophthalmia]. Graefes Arch Clin Exp Ophthalmol 1975;193:229–243.

53. Chan CC, Palestine AG, Nussenblatt RB, et al. Anti-retinal auto-antibodies in Vogt-Koyanagi-Harada syndrome, Behçet's disease, and sympathetic ophthalmia. Ophthalmology 1985;92:1025–1028.

54. Wong VG, Anderson R, O'Brien PJ. Sympathetic ophthalmia and lymphocyte transformation. Am J Ophthalmol 1971;72:960–966.

55. Marak GE Jr, Font RL, Johnson MC, Alepa FP. Lymphocyte-stimulating activity of ocular tissues in sympathetic ophthalmia. Invest Ophthalmol 1971;10:770–774.

56. Kincses E, Torok M. Study on cellular immune response after complicated cataract operations and in sympathetic ophthalmia. Graefes Arch Clin Exp Ophthalmol 1977;204:149–152.

57. Aronson SB, Hogan MJ, Zweigart P. Homoimmune uveitis in the guinea pig. I. General concepts of auto- and homoimmunity, methods, and manifestations. Arch Ophthalmol 1963;69:105–109.

58. Collins RC. Further experimental studies on sympathetic ophthalmia. Am J Ophthalmol 1953;36:150–161.

59. Lubin JR, Albert DM, Weinstein M. Sixty-five years of sympathetic ophthalmia. A clinicopathologic review of 105 cases (1913–1978). Ophthalmology 1980;87:109–121.

60. Mahoney BP. Rheumatologic Disease. In BH Blaustein (ed), Ocular Manifestations of Systemic Disease. New York: Churchill Livingstone, 1994;61–80.

61. Abel GS. Uveitis. In DK Roberts, JE Terry (eds), Ocular Disease: Diagnosis and Treatment. Boston: Butterworth–Heinemann, 1996;533.

62. Fox R, Calin A, Gerber RC, Gibson D. The chronicity of symptoms and disability in Reiter's syndrome. An analysis of 131 consecutive patients. Ann Intern Med 1979;91:190–193.

63. Csonka GW. The course of Reiter's syndrome. Br Med J 1958;1:1088–1090.

64. Holland EJ. Reiter's Syndrome. In DH Gold, TA Weingeist (eds), The Eye in Systemic Disease. Philadelphia: Lippincott, 1990;56–57.

65. Godfrey WA. Acute Anterior Uveitis. In W Tasman, EA Jaeger (eds), Duane's Ophthalmology on CD-ROM. Philadelphia: Lippincott–Raven, 1997.

66. Miller-Blair DJ, Tsuchiya N, Yamaguchi A, et al. Immunologic mechanisms in common rheumatologic diseases. Clin Orthop 1996;326:43–54.

67. Calin A. Reiter's Syndrome. In A Calin (ed), Spondyloarthropathies. Orlando, FL: Grune & Stratton, 1984;119.

68. Feltkamp TE, Khan MA, Lopez de Castro JA. The pathogenetic role of HLA-B27. Immunol Today 1996;17:5–7.

69. Schachter J. Isolation of *Bedsoniae* from human arthritis and abortion tissues. Am J Ophthalmol 1967;63(suppl):1082–1086.

70. Ostler HB, Schachter J, Dawson CR. Ocular infection of rabbits with a *Bedsonia* isolated from a patient with Reiter's syndrome. Invest Ophthalmol Vis Sci 1970;9:256–262.

71. Hardin JG, Longenecker GL. Handbook of Drug Therapy in Rheumatic Disease: Pharmacology and Clinical Aspects. Boston: Little, Brown, 1992;197.

72. Calin A. A placebo-controlled, cross-over study of azathioprine in Reiter's syndrome. Ann Rheum Dis 1986;45:653–655.

73. Lally EV, Ho G Jr. A review of methotrexate therapy in Reiter syndrome. Semin Arthritis Rheum 1985;15:139–145.

74. Kimura SJ, Hogan MJ, O'Connor GR, Epstein WV. Uveitis and joint diseases: a review of 191 cases. Trans Am Ophthalmol Soc 1966;64:291–310.

75. Rahi AH. HLA and eye disease. Br J Ophthalmol 1979;63:283–292.

76. Saari R, Lahti R, Saari KM, et al. Frequency of rheumatic diseases in patients with acute anterior uveitis. Scand J Rheumatol 1982;11:121–123.

77. Friedlaender MH. Allergy and Immunology of the Eye (2nd ed). New York: Raven Press, 1992;224.

78. Ebringer A. The cross-tolerance hypothesis, HLA-B27 and ankylosing spondylitis. Br J Rheumatol 1983;22(4 suppl 2):53–66.

79. Ebringer A, Ahmadi K, Fielder M, et al. Molecular mimicry: the geographical distribution of immune responses to *Klebsiella* in ankylosing spondylitis and its relevance to therapy. Clin Rheumatol 1996;15(suppl 1):57–61.

80. Maksymowych WP, Jhangri GS, Gorodezky C, et al. The LMP2 polymorphism is associated with susceptibility to acute anterior uveitis in HLA-B27 positive juvenile and adult Mexican subjects with ankylosing spondylitis. Ann Rheum Dis 1997;56:488–492.

81. Wendling D, Racadot E, Toussirot E, Wijdenes J. Combination therapy of anti-CD4 and anti-IL-6 monoclonal antibodies in a case of severe spondyloarthropathy [letter]. Br J Rheumatol 1996;35:1330.

82. Jabs DA. Ocular Manifestations of the Rheumatic Diseases. In W Tasman, EA Jaeger (eds), Duane's Clinical Ophthalmology. Philadelphia: Lippincott–Raven, 1996;3.

83. Harris ED. Rheumatoid Arthritis: The Clinical Spectrum. In WN Kelley (ed), Textbook of Rheumatology (2nd ed). Philadelphia: Saunders, 1985;915–950.

84. Hedfors E, Klareskog L, Lindblad S, et al. Phenotypic characterization of cells within subcutaneous rheumatoid nodules. Arthritis Rheum 1983;26:1333–1339.

85. Mahoney BP. Rheumatologic Disease. In BH Blaustein (ed), Ocular Manifestations of Systemic Disease. New York: Churchill Livingstone, 1994;65.

86. McGavin DD, Williamson J, Forrester JV, et al. Episcleritis and scleritis. A study of their clinical manifestations and their association with rheumatoid arthritis. Br J Ophthalmol 1976;60:192–226.

87. Williamson J. Incidence of eye disease in cases of connective tissue disease. Trans Ophthalmol Soc UK 1974;94:742–752.

88. Foster CS, Forstot SL, Wilson LA. Mortality rate in rheumatoid arthritis patients developing necrotizing scleritis or peripheral ulcerative keratitis. Ophthalmology 1984;91:1253–1263.

89. Giordano N, D'Ettorre M, Biasi G, et al. Retinal vasculitis in rheumatoid arthritis: an angiographic study. Clin Exp Rheumatol 1990;8:121–125.

90. Schaller J, Kupfer C, Wedgewood RJ. Iridocyclitis in juvenile rheumatoid arthritis. Pediatrics 1969;44:92–100.

91. Johnson PM, Watkins J, Holborow EJ. Anti-globulin production to altered IgG in rheumatoid arthritis. Lancet 1975;1:611–614.

92. Bell C, Talal N, Schur PH. Antibodies to DNA in patients with rheumatoid arthritis and juvenile rheumatoid arthritis. Arthritis Rheum 1975;18:535–540.

93. Andriopoulos NA, Mestecky J, Miller EJ, Bennett JC. Antibodies to human native and denatured collagens in synovial fluids of patients with rheumatoid arthritis. Clin Immunol Immunopathol 1976;6:209–212.

94. Thonar EJ, Sweet MB. Cellular hypersensitivity in rheumatoid arthritis, ankylosing spondylitis, and anterior nongranulomatous uveitis.Arthritis Rheum 1976;19:539–544.

95. Person DA, Sharp JT, Lidsky MD. The cytotoxicity of leukocytes and lymphocytes from patients with rheumatoid arthritis for synovial cells. J Clin Invest 1976;58:690–698.

96. McDermott M, McDevitt H. The immunogenetics of rheumatic diseases. Bull Rheum Dis 1988;38:1–10.

97. Friedlaender MH. Allergy and Immunology of the Eye (2nd ed). New York: Raven Press, 1992;228.

98. Karameris A, Gorgoulis V, Iliopoulos A, et al. Detection of the Epstein-Barr viral genome by an in situ hybridization method in salivary gland biopsies from patients with secondary Sjögren's syndrome. Clin Exp Rheumatol 1992;10:327–332.

99. Jansson E, Makisara P, Tuuri S. *Mycoplasma* antibodies in rheumatoid arthritis. Scand J Rheumatol 1975;4:165–168.

100. McDowell TL, Symons JA, Ploski R, et al. A genetic association between juvenile rheumatoid arthritis and a novel interleukin-1 alpha polymorphism. Arthritis Rheum 1995;38:221–228.

101. Ruddy S. The Management of Rheumatoid Arthritis. In WN Kelley (ed), Textbook of Rheumatology (2nd ed). Philadelphia: Saunders, 1985;950–966.

102. Finbloom DS, Silver K, Newsome DA, Gunkel R. Comparison of hydroxychloroquine and chloroquine use and the development of retinal toxicity. J Rheumatol 1985;12:692–694.

103. Hill JC. Slow-release artificial tear inserts in the treatment of dry eyes in patients with rheumatoid arthritis. Br J Ophthalmol 1989;73:151–154.

104. Kagnoff MF. Oral tolerance: mechanisms and possible role in inflammatory joint diseases. Baillieres Clin Rheumatol 1996;10:41–54.

105. Kingsley G, Lanchbury J, Panayi G. Immunotherapy in rheumatic disease: an idea whose time has come—or gone? Immunol Today 1996;17:9–12.
106. Abel GS. Uveitis. In DK Roberts, JE Terry (eds), Ocular Disease: Diagnosis and Treatment. Boston: Butterworth–Heinemann, 1996;540.
107. Nussenblatt RB, Whitcup SM, Palestine AG. Uveitis. Fundamentals and Clinical Practice (2nd ed). St. Louis: Mosby, 1996;335.
108. Chajek T, Fainaru M. Behçet's disease. Report of 41 cases and a review of the literature. Medicine 1975;54:179–196.
109. Imai Y. The prognosis on Behçet's disease under long period of observation. Nippon Ganka Gakkai Zasshi 1970;74:1118–1120.
110. Gamble CN, Wiesner KB, Shapiro RF, Boyer WJ. The immune complex pathogenesis of glomerulonephritis and pulmonary vasculitis in Behçet's disease. Am J Med 1979;66:1031–1039.
111. Levinsky RJ, Lehner T. Circulating soluble immune complexes in recurrent oral ulceration and Behçet's syndrome. Clin Exp Immunol 1978;32:193–198.
112. Kasp E, Graham EM, Stanford MR, et al. Retinal Autoimmunity and Circulating Immune Complexes in Ocular Behçet's Disease. In T Lehner, CG Barnes (eds), Recent Advances in Behçet's Disease. London: Royal Society of Medicine Services, 1986.
113. Mizuki N, Inoko H, Ohno S. Pathogenic gene responsible for the predisposition of Behçet's disease. Int Rev Immunol 1997;14:33–48.
114. Poulter LW, Lehner T, Duke O. Immunohistological Investigation of Recurrent Oral Ulcers and Behçet's Disease. In T Lehner, CG Barnes (eds), Recent Advances in Behçet's Disease. London: Royal Society of Medicine Services, 1986.
115. Charteris DG, Champ C, Rosenthal AR, Lightman SL. Behçet's disease: activated T lymphocytes in retinal perivasculitis. Br J Ophthalmol 1992;76:499–501.
116. Valesini G, Pivetti-Pezzi P, Mastrandrea F, et al. Evaluation of T cell subsets in Behçet's syndrome using anti-T cell monoclonal antibodies. Clin Exp Immunol 1985;60:55–60.
117. Ohno S, Kato F, Matsuda H, et al. Studies on spontaneous production of gamma-interferon in Behçet's disease. Ophthalmologica 1982;185:187–192.
118. BenEzra D, Maftzir G, Kalichman I, Barak V. Serum levels of interleukin-2 receptor in ocular Behçet's disease. Am J Ophthalmol 1993;115:26–30.
119. Charteris DG, Barton K, McCartney AC, Lightman SL. CD4+ lymphocyte involvement in ocular Behçet's disease. Autoimmunity 1992;12:201–206.
120. Yamamoto JH, Minami M, Inaba G, et al. Cellular autoimmunity to retinal specific antigens in patients with Behçet's disease. Br J Ophthalmol 1993;77: 584–589.
121. Sakane T. New perspective on Behçet's disease. Int Rev Immunol 1997;14: 89–96.
122. Lehner T. The role of heat shock protein, microbial and autoimmune agents in the aetiology of Behçet's disease. Int Rev Immunol 1997;14:21–32.
123. Kotter I, Durk H, Eckstein A, et al. Erosive arthritis and posterior uveitis in Behçet's disease: treatment with interferon alpha and interferon gamma. Clin Exp Rheumatol 1996;14:313–315.

124. Jabs DA. The Rheumatic Diseases. In S Ryna (ed), The Retina (vol 2). St. Louis: Mosby, 1989;457–480.

125. Stahl NI, Klippel JH, Decker JL. Fever in systemic lupus erythematosus. Am J Med 1979;67:935–940.

126. Schur PH. Clinical Features of Systemic Lupus Erythematosus. In WN Kelley (ed), Textbook of Rheumatology (4th ed). Philadelphia: Saunders, 1993;1017.

127. Nussenblatt RB, Tabbara KF. Autoimmune Diseases. In KF Tabbara, RB Nussenblatt (eds), Posterior Uveitis: Diagnosis and Management. Boston: Butterworth–Heinemann, 1994;87.

128. Mahoney BP. Rheumatologic Disease. In BH Blaustein (ed), Ocular Manifestations of Systemic Disease. New York: Churchill Livingstone, 1994;67.

129. Rosenstein ED, Sobelman J, Kramer N. Isolated, pupil-sparing third nerve palsy as initial manifestation of systemic lupus erythematosus. J Clin Neuroophthalmol 1989;9:285–288.

130. Rosenbaum JT. Systemic Lupus Erythematosus. In FT Fraunfelder, FH Roy (eds), Current Ocular Therapy. Philadelphia: Saunders, 1990;206.

131. Jabs DA, Fine SL, Hochberg MC, et al. Severe retinal vaso-occlusive disease in systemic lupus erythematosus. Arch Ophthalmol 1986;104:558–563.

132. Tsokos GC, Kovacs B, Liossis SN. Lymphocytes, cytokines, inflammation, and immune trafficking. Curr Opin Rheumatol 1997;9:380–386.

133. Suzuki N, Mihara S, Sakane T. Development of pathogenic anti-DNA antibodies in patients with systemic lupus erythematosus. FASEB J 1997;11:1033–1038.

134. Nash PD, Opas M, Michalak M. Calreticulin not just another calcium-binding protein. Mol Cell Biochem 1994;135:71–78.

135. Eggleton P, Reid KB, Kishore U, Sontheimer RD. Clinical relevance of calreticulin in systemic lupus erythematosus. Lupus 1997;6:564–571.

136. Bengtsson A, Blomberg J, Nived O, et al. Selective antibody reactivity with peptides from human endogenous retroviruses and nonviral poly(amino acids) in patients with systemic lupus erythematosus. Arthritis Rheum 1996;39:1654–1663.

137. Friedlaender MH. Allergy and Immunology of the Eye (2nd ed). New York: Raven Press, 1992;237.

138. Tamura N, Sekigawa I, Hashimoto H, et al. Syncytial cell formation in vivo by type C retroviral particles in the systemic lupus erythematosus (SLE) lung. Clin Exp Immunol 1997;107:474–479.

139. Burlingame RW. The clinical utility of antihistone antibodies. Autoantibodies reactive with chromatin in systemic lupus erythematosus and drug-induced lupus. Clin Lab Med 1997;17:367–378.

140. Hannouche D, Korobelnik JF, Cochereau I, et al. Systemic lupus erythematosus with choroidopathy and serous retinal detachment. Int Ophthalmol 1995;19:125–127.

141. Fox RI, Maruyama T. Pathogenesis and treatment of Sjögren's syndrome. Curr Opin Rheumatol 1997;9:393–399.

142. Friedlaender MH. Allergy and Immunology of the Eye (2nd ed). New York: Raven Press, 1992;241.

143. Mahoney BP. Rheumatologic Disease. In BH Blaustein (ed), Ocular Manifestations of Systemic Disease. New York: Churchill Livingstone, 1994;70.

144. Price EJ, Venables PJ. The etiopathogenesis of Sjögren's syndrome. Semin Arthritis Rheum 1995;25:117–133.

145. Fox RI. Sjögren's syndrome. Controversies and progress. Clin Lab Med 1997;17:431–444.

146. Haneji N, Nakamura T, Takio K, et al. Identification of alpha-fodrin as a candidate autoantigen in primary Sjögren's syndrome. Science 1997;276:604–607.

147. Maddison PJ. Dry eyes: autoimmunity and relationship to other systemic disease. Trans Ophthalmol Soc UK 1985;104:458–461.

148. Nakamura S, Ikebe-Hiroki A, Shinohara M, et al. An association between salivary gland disease and serological abnormalities in Sjögren's syndrome. J Oral Pathol Med 1997;26:426–430.

149. Kumagai S, Kanagawa S, Morinobu A, et al. Association of a new allele of the TAP2 gene, TAP2*Bky2 (Val577), with susceptibility to Sjögren's syndrome. Arthritis Rheum 1997;40:1685–1692.

150. Griffith KJ, Chan EK, Lung CC, et al. Molecular cloning of a novel 97-kd Golgi complex autoantigen associated with Sjögren's syndrome. Arthritis Rheum 1997;40:1693–1702.

151. Bacman S, Leiros CP, Sterin-Borda L, et al. Autoantibodies against lacrimal gland M_3 muscarinic acetylcholine receptors in patients with primary Sjögren's syndrome. Invest Ophthalmol Vis Sci 1998;39:151–156.

152. Kruize AA, Smeenk RJ, Kater L. Diagnostic criteria and immunopathogenesis of Sjögren's syndrome: implications for therapy. Immunol Today 1995;16:557–559.

153. Fox RI, Kang HI, Ando D, et al. Cytokine mRNA expression in salivary gland biopsies of Sjögren's syndrome. J Immunol 1994;152:5532–5539.

154. Ogawa N, Ohashi H. [Study of apoptosis in Sjögren's syndrome]. Rinsho Byori 1997;45:643–648.

155. Lynch DH, Ramsdell F, Alderson MR. Fas and FasL in the homeostatic regulation of immune responses. Immunol Today 1995;16:569–574.

156. Humphreys-Beher MG. Animal models for autoimmune disease-associated xerostomia and xerophthalmia. Adv Dent Res 1996;10:73–75.

157. Haneji N, Hamano H, Yanagi K, Hayashi Y. A new animal model for primary Sjögren's syndrome in NFS/sld mutant mice. J Immunol 1994;153:2769–2777.

158. Mircheff AK, Warren DW, Wood RL. Hormonal support of lacrimal function, primary lacrimal deficiency, autoimmunity, and peripheral tolerance in the lacrimal gland. Ocul Immunol Inflamm 1996;4:145–172.

159. Verheul HA, Verveld M, Hoefakker S, Schuurs AH. Effects of ethynylestradiol on the course of spontaneous autoimmune disease in NZB/W and NOD mice. Immunopharmacol Immunotoxicol 1995;17:163–180.

160. Hayashi Y, Haneji N, Hamano H, Yanagi K. Transfer of Sjögren's syndrome-like autoimmune lesions into SCID mice and prevention of lesions by anti-CD4 and anti-T cell receptor antibody treatment. Eur J Immunol 1994;24:2826–2831.

161. Spiera H, Asbell PA, Simpson DM. Botulinum toxin increases tearing in patients with Sjögren's syndrome: a preliminary report. J Rheumatol 1997;24:1842–1843.

162. Ferraccioli GF, Salaffi F, De Vita S, et al. Interferon alpha-2 (IFN-α2) increases lacrimal and salivary function in Sjögren's syndrome patients. Preliminary results of an open pilot trial versus OH-chloroquine. Clin Exp Rheumatol 1996;14:367–371.

163. Nussenblatt RB, Whitcup SM, Palestine AG. Uveitis. Fundamentals and Clinical Practice (2nd ed). St. Louis: Mosby, 1996;313.

164. Moorthy RS, Inomata H, Rao NA. Vogt-Koyanagi-Harada syndrome. Surv Ophthalmol 1995;39:265–292.

165. Ohno S, Minakawa R, Matsuda H. Clinical studies of Vogt-Koyanagi-Harada's disease. Jpn J Ophthalmol 1988;32:334–343.

166. Kishi A, Nao-i N, Sawada A. Ultrasound biomicroscopic findings of acute angle-closure glaucoma in Vogt-Koyanagi-Harada syndrome. Am J Ophthalmol 1996;122:735–737.

167. Nussenblatt RB, Tabbara KF. Autoimmune Diseases. In KF Tabbara, RB Nussenblatt (eds), Posterior Uveitis: Diagnosis and Management. Boston: Butterworth–Heinemann, 1994;90.

168. Weisz JM, Holland GN, Roer LN, et al. Association between Vogt-Koyanagi-Harada syndrome and HLA-DR1 and -DR4 in Hispanic patients living in southern California. Ophthalmology 1995;102:1012–1015.

169. Kahn M, Pepose JS, Green WR, et al. Immunocytologic findings in a case of Vogt-Koyanagi-Harada syndrome. Ophthalmology 1993;100:1191–1198.

170. Friedenwald JS, McKee KM. A filter-passing agent as a cause in endophthalmitis. Am J Ophthalmol 1938;21:723–738.

171. Liu T, Sun SM. [Peripheral lymphocyte subsets in patients with Vogt-Koyanagi-Harada syndrome (VKH)]. Chung Hua Yen Ko Tsa Chih 1993;29:138–140.

172. Okubo K, Kurimoto S, Okubo K, et al. Surface markers of peripheral blood lymphocytes in Vogt-Koyanagi-Harada disease. J Clin Lab Immunol 1985;17:49–52.

173. Yuasa T, Murai Y, Hoki T, Mimura Y. [Lymphocyte transformation test and migration inhibition test of macrophages in Vogt-Koyanagi-Harada's syndrome (author's transl)]. Nippon Ganka Gakkai Zasshi 1973;77:1652–1657.

174. Maezawa N, Yano A, Taniguchi M, Kojima S. The role of cytotoxic T lymphocytes in the pathogenesis of Vogt-Koyanagi-Harada disease. Ophthalmologica 1982;185:179–186.

175. Sugita S, Sagawa K, Mochizuki M, et al. Melanocyte lysis by cytotoxic T lymphocytes recognizing the MART-1 melanoma antigen in HLA-A2 patients with Vogt-Koyanagi-Harada disease. Int Immunol 1996;8:799–803.

176. Nakamura S, Nakazawa M, Yoshioka M, et al. Melanin-laden macrophages in cerebrospinal fluid in Vogt-Koyanagi-Harada syndrome. Arch Ophthalmol 1996;114:1184–1188.

177. Nussenblatt RB, Gery I, Ballintine EJ, Wacker WB. Cellular immune responsiveness of uveitis patients to retinal S-antigen. Am J Ophthalmol 1980;89:173–179.

178. Norose K, Yano A, Wang XC, et al. Dominance of activated T-cells and interleukin-6 in aqueous humor in Vogt-Koyanagi-Harada disease. Invest Ophthalmol Vis Sci 1994;35:33–39.

179. Kumano Y, Nagato T, Kurihara K, et al. Hyperimmunoglobulinemia D in idiopathic retinal vasculitis. Graefes Arch Clin Exp Ophthalmol 1997; 235:372–378.

180. Nussenblatt RB, Palestine AG, Chan CC. Cyclosporin A therapy in the treatment of intraocular inflammatory disease resistant to systemic corticosteroids and cytotoxic agents. Am J Ophthalmol 1983;96:275–282.

181. Ishioka M, Ohno S, Nakamura S, et al. FK506 treatment of noninfectious uveitis. Am J Ophthalmol 1994;118:723–729.

182. Abel GS. Uveitis. In DK Roberts, JE Terry (eds), Ocular Disease: Diagnosis and Treatment. Boston: Butterworth–Heinemann, 1996;541.

183. Newman LS, Rose CS, Maier LA. Sarcoidosis. N Engl J Med 1997;336: 1224–1234.

184. Nussenblatt RB, Whitcup SM, Palestine AG. Uveitis. Fundamentals and Clinical Practice (2nd ed). St. Louis: Mosby, 1996;290.

185. Friedlaender MH. Allergy and Immunology of the Eye (2nd ed). New York: Raven Press, 1992;265.

186. Obenauf CD, Shaw HE, Sydnor CF, Klintworth GK. Sarcoidosis and its ophthalmic manifestations. Am J Ophthalmol 1978;86:648–655.

187. Jabs DA, Johns CJ. Ocular involvement in chronic sarcoidosis. Am J Ophthalmol 1986;102:297–301.

188. Spalton DJ, Sanders MD. Fundus changes in histologically confirmed sarcoidosis. Br J Ophthalmol 1981;65:348–358.

189. Grunewald J, Janson CH, Eklund A, et al. Restricted V alpha 2.3 gene usage by CD4+ T lymphocytes in bronchoalveolar lavage fluid from sarcoidosis patients correlates with HLA-DR3. Eur J Immunol 1992;22:129–135.

190. Ishihara M, Ohno S. Genetic influences on sarcoidosis. Eye 1997;11:155–161.

191. Burke WM, Keogh A, Maloney PJ, et al. Transmission of sarcoidosis via cardiac transplantation. Lancet 1990;336:1579.

192. Heyll A, Meckenstock G, Aul C, et al. Possible transmission of sarcoidosis via allogeneic bone marrow transplantation. Bone Marrow Transplant 1994;14:161–164.

193. Saboor SA, Johnson NM, McFadden J. Detection of mycobacterial DNA in sarcoidosis and tuberculosis with polymerase chain reaction. Lancet 1992;339:1012–1015.

194. Tamura N, Suzuki K, Iwase A, et al. [Retroviral infection as a putative pathogen for sarcoidosis]. Nippon Rinsho 1994;52:1503–1507.

195. Steffan M, Petersen J, Oldigs M, et al. Increased secretion of tumor necrosis factor-alpha, interleukin-1-beta, and interleukin-6 by alveolar macrophages from patients with sarcoidosis. J Allergy Clin Immunol 1993;91:939–949.

196. Hirschhorn K, Schreibman RR, Bach FH, Siltzbach LE. In vitro studies of lymphocytes from patients with sarcoidosis and lymphoproliferative disease. Lancet 1964;2:842–843.

197. Tabbara KF. Other Disorders. In KF Tabbara, RB Nussenblatt (eds), Posterior Uveitis: Diagnosis and Management. Boston: Butterworth–Heinemann, 1994;116.

198. Smith RJ, Manche EE, Mondino BJ. Ocular Cicatricial Pemphigoid and Ocular Manifestations of Pemphigus Vulgaris. In G Smolin (ed), International Ophthalmology Clinics: Ocular Manifestations of Dermatologic Disorders. Philadelphia: Lippincott–Raven, 1997;37:63–75.

199. Seamone CD, Jackson WB. Immunology of the External Eye. In W Tasman, EA Jaeger (eds), Duane's Ophthalmology on CD-ROM. Philadelphia: Lippincott–Raven, 1997.

200. Mondino BJ, Brown SI. Ocular cicatricial pemphigoid. Ophthalmology 1981;88:95–100.

201. Foster CS. Immunologic Disorders of the Conjunctiva, Cornea, and Sclera. In DM Albert, FA Jakobiec (eds), Principles and Practice of Ophthalmology. Philadelphia: Saunders, 1994;197.

202. Foster CS. Cicatricial pemphigoid. Trans Am Ophthalmol Soc 1986;84:527–663.

203. Mondino BJ. Cicatricial pemphigoid and erythema multiforme. Ophthalmology 1990;97:939–952.

204. Mondino BJ, Ross AN, Rabin BS, Brown SI. Autoimmune phenomena in ocular cicatricial pemphigoid. Am J Ophthalmol 1977;83:443–450.

205. Hsu R, Lazarova Z, Yee C, Yancey KB. Noncomplement fixing, IgG4 autoantibodies predominate in patients with anti-epiligrin cicatricial pemphigoid. J Invest Dermatol 1997;109:557–561.

206. Chan LS, Majmudar AA, Tran HH, et al. Laminin-6 and laminin-5 are recognized by autoantibodies in a subset of cicatricial pemphigoid. J Invest Dermatol 1997;108:848–853.

207. Ghohestani RF, Nicolas JF, Rousselle P, Claudy AL. Identification of a 168-kDa mucosal antigen in a subset of patients with cicatricial pemphigoid. J Invest Dermatol 1996;107:136–139.

208. Tyagi S, Bhol K, Natarajan K, et al. Ocular cicatricial pemphigoid antigen: partial sequence and biochemical characterization. Proc Natl Acad Sci U S A 1996;93:14714–14719.

209. Balding SD, Prost C, Diaz LA, et al. Cicatricial pemphigoid autoantibodies react with multiple sites on the BP180 extracellular domain. J Invest Dermatol 1996;106:141–146.

210. Bedane C, McMillan JR, Balding SD, et al. Bullous pemphigoid and cicatricial pemphigoid autoantibodies react with ultrastructurally separable epitopes on the BP180 ectodomain: evidence that BP180 spans the lamina lucida. J Invest Dermatol 1997;108:901–907.

211. Ahmed AR, Foster S, Zaltas M, et al. Association of DQw7 (DQB1*0301) with ocular cicatricial pemphigoid. Proc Natl Acad Sci U S A 1991;88:11579–11582.

212. Hirst LW, Werblin T, Novak M, et al. Drug-induced cicatrizing conjunctivitis simulating ocular pemphigoid. Cornea 1982;1:121–128.

213. Fern AI, Jay JL, Young H, MacKie R. Dapsone therapy for the acute inflammatory phase of ocular pemphigoid. Br J Ophthalmol 1992;76:332–335.

CHAPTER 6

Ocular Tumor Immunology

Based upon observations on 48 cases of retinoblastoma and published reports, the hypothesis is developed that retinoblastoma is a cancer caused by two mutational events. In the dominantly inherited form, one mutation is inherited via the germinal cells and the second occurs in somatic cells. In the non-hereditary form, both mutations occur in somatic cells. [*]

Normal cells become cancerous by undergoing a process called *malignant transformation* that enables them to grow and divide in an unregulated manner. It is the bane of cancer diagnosis that such a cell and its progeny undergo nearly 30 population doublings to produce 10^9 cells weighing 1 g before the tumor can be detected clinically. How long this process takes depends on the tissue and can range from 3 months to several years. Although certain ocular tumors can be detected when somewhat smaller, the fact remains that a significant tumor load already exists at the time of diagnosis and the tumor has already completed a major portion of its life cycle.[1]

An initial tumor is referred to as a *primary tumor*. Although all cells of such a tumor may have been derived from a single transformed cell, they are far from identical. Heterogeneity in a tumor cell population develops as a result of multiple mutations that develop independently in different cells. These mutations account for tumor cells' variable ability to break free and metastasize and also influence their susceptibility to chemotherapeutic agents. Cells that have developed metastatic potential elaborate cell-surface receptors that promote their adhesion to basement membrane and connective tissue ligands and also secrete proteases that promote their passage through the extracellular matrix and into the circulation.

---

[*]From Alfred G. Knudson Jr.'s exposition of what has come to be called the *two-hit hypothesis* for retinoblastoma formation (from Mutation and cancer: statistical study of retinoblastoma. *Proc Natl Acad Sci U S A* 1971;68:820–823).

Once in the circulation, tumor cells tend to aggregate into clumps. These clumps may be attacked by circulating natural killer (NK) cells, which play a role in immune surveillance. Platelets also adhere to these tumor clumps, which unfortunately protects them from immune attack and enhances their ability to implant on a vessel wall and enter underlying tissues to produce a metastatic deposit. Adhesion molecules on the tumor cells also play a role in implantation, and it is likely that such molecules bind to ligands that may be preferentially expressed in one target organ. For example, ocular melanomas preferentially metastasize to the liver while prostatic carcinoma preferentially spreads to the bones. Clearly, circulatory and lymphoid drainage dynamics also play a role. A summary of the various steps in tumor cell growth and metastasis is shown in Figure 6.1.

This chapter deals specifically with two intraocular tumors: melanoma, which is the most common primary intraocular malignancy, and retinoblastoma, which is the most common intraocular childhood malignancy. As we will see, tumor-specific antigens are present on cells of both of these tumors, and their immune-mediated destruction has been demonstrated in vitro. The location of these tumors intraocularly, however, places them in an immune-privileged site where the full immune system arsenal is unavailable to fight them. We first discuss how the unique intraocular immune environment affects the immune system's ability to combat intraocular tumors, and then specifically discuss these tumors and their epidemiology, clinical features, pathogenesis, and treatment.

Intraocular Regulation of Antitumor Immunity

Role of Natural Killer Cells

NK cells play an important role in eliminating tumor cells. NK cell affinity for tumor cells is thought to relate to their ability to specifically recognize and bind to cells such as tumor cells that either fail to express, or express very low levels of, class I antigens. In addition to binding directly to tumor cells, NK cells can also lyse tumor cells by antibody-dependent cellular cytotoxicity. An important constituent in aqueous humor that influences intraocular immune function is transforming growth factor–beta (TGF-β). As discussed in Chapter 2, TGF-β inhibits various immune processes such as lymphocyte activation and proliferation and it plays a major role in mediating the phenomenon of anterior chamber–associated immune deviation (ACAID). TGF-β also inhibits NK cell activity.[2] Interestingly, TGF-β was shown to reduce major histocompatibility complex (MHC) class I expression on human uveal melanoma cells, thus increasing their susceptibility to NK-mediated lysis.[3] A second aqueous humor factor called *natural killer inhibitory factor* also has profound inhibitory effects on NK-mediated lysis of tumor cells in vitro.[4] Specifically, it inhibits the release of NK cytolytic

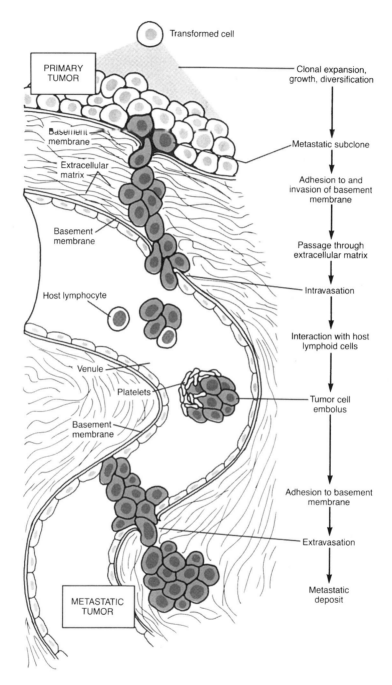

FIGURE 6.1. The metastatic cascade. Illustration of the sequential steps involved in the hematogenous spread of a tumor. (Reprinted with permission from RS Cotran, V Kumar, SL Robbins. Robbins' Pathologic Basis of Disease [5th ed]. Philadelphia: Saunders, 1994;277.)

factors but does not appear to block the binding of NK cells to tumor cells.[5] Although it is reasonable to suggest that NK-mediated lysis of intraocular tumors is compromised as a result of the action of the above-mentioned factors, this suggestion presupposes that NK cells are involved in the elimination of intraocular tumors. Immunohistochemical studies of human uveal melanomas demonstrated the presence of infiltrating NK cells,[6,7] and one of these studies showed that it was the predominant infiltrating immune cell.[7] Furthermore, Niederkorn showed that NK-sensitive RMA-S murine lymphoma cells and NK-sensitive OCM-3 human uveal melanoma cells were rejected by NK cells following subcutaneous transplantation, yet grew progressively when the same or much lower numbers of tumor cells were transplanted intracamerally.[5] Therefore, the intraocular environment appears to allow tumors to escape immune surveillance and destruction by NK cells.

Role of Anterior Chamber–Associated Immune Deviation

Recall from Chapter 2 that ACAID refers to the unique immune-response modulation that occurs in reaction to antigens in the anterior chamber. Specifically, antigen-directed, delayed-type hypersensitivity (DTH) and complement-fixing antibodies are suppressed systemically (as well as locally in response to immunosuppressive factors in the aqueous humor). A host of antigens can elicit ACAID, including herpes simplex virus antigen, retinal S antigen, soluble proteinaceous antigens, and certain tumor antigens such as melanoma-associated antigens. Histoincompatible P815 mastocytoma cells elicit ACAID when injected into BALB/c mice, though mutagenized P815 cells, as well as other tumor antigens such as a mutagenized clone of melanoma cells and certain ultraviolet-induced or SV-40 large T antigen–bearing tumors, did not.[8–10] Tumors that were rejected elicited vigorous DTH and cytotoxic T cell responses. Evidence suggests that ACAID-like immune modulation also occurs in response to antigens, such as retinal allografts, placed into either the vitreous cavity or the subretinal region.[11] Clearly, intraocular tumors evade immune surveillance in part as a result of ACAID, though particularly immunogenic tumor-specific antigens can circumvent ACAID. This may account for the spontaneous regression that occurs in certain intraocular tumors such as retinoblastoma.

Role of T Cells

Lymphocytes have been observed in a minority of ocular tumors, particularly uveal melanomas. When present, they are referred to as *tumor-infiltrating lymphocytes* (TILs) and comprise NK cells[7] and T lymphocytes[12] in varying numbers, depending on the tumor. These cells were shown to play a role in the destruction of intraocular tumors in animals, as alluded to with regard to NK cells. In mice injected with highly immunogenic UV-induced fibrosarcoma cells, subsequent tumors into which TILs infiltrated were destroyed.[13] These tumors contained TILs consisting of both CD4+ helper and CD8+ cytotoxic cells. In mice with uveal melanomas, TILs were shown to consist initially of primarily CD4+ cells, but CD8+ cytotoxic cells predominated during the resolution phase.[14] Most interestingly, destruction of the tumor occurred without ancillary damage to other ocular structures, suggesting that antitumor DTH was not taking place. Immunohistochemical and cytotoxicity assay results all suggested that cytotoxic T cells were responsible for tumor resolution. Furthermore, adoptive transfer of TILs into immunocompromised animals resulted in the elimination of their intraocular tumor. When tested peripherally, animals with fibrosarcoma tumors showed strong DTH in addition to cytotoxic responses to tumor antigens.

The fact that cytotoxic T cells can lyse intraocular tumor cells implies that the tumor cells express tumor antigens. Numerous tumor antigens have been described for cutaneous melanoma, including the family of genes known as *melanoma antigen genes* (MAGE), as well as those encoded by the tyrosinase gene (tyrosinase converts tyrosine to dihydroxyphenylalanine, or DOPA, which is a precursor of melanin). Less than 10% of human uveal tumors express MAGE antigens, though expression of tyrosinase is high.[15] Retinoblastomas have been shown to express rhodopsin, S antigen, and preproenkephalin.

It has been difficult to come to a consensus regarding whether the presence of TILs in intraocular human tumors is a good prognostic sign.[16–18] Although it would seem logical to assume, based on the animal data, that the infiltration of human intraocular tumors by immune cells is a positive development, the evidence is equivocal.[5] This may be a result, in part, of differences in tumor antigenicity. This is supported by the evidence in mice that the antigens expressed on semiallogeneic P815 mastocytoma cells are insufficient to trigger full differentiation of TILs into functioning cytotoxic T cells.[19]

Ocular Melanoma

Ocular melanomas develop most commonly in the uveal tract, with ciliary body and choroidal melanomas being more common and more life threatening than iris melanomas. Choroidal melanomas are the most frequent type, followed by ciliary body and iris melanomas, respectively. The cells in the uvea that develop into melanomas are melanocytes and are developmentally derived from the neural crest. In the iris, the melanocytes are found lining the anterior surface of the stroma together with fibroblasts and within the anterior stromal sheet in a homogeneous ground substance containing some collagen fibers. Ciliary body melanocytes are found in the interstices between the muscle bundles, being especially numerous toward the sclera. In the choroid, large, flat melanocytes are found between and within the connective tissue lamellae. The pigmented epithelia in the iris, ciliary body, and retina are derived as an outgrowth of the developing neural tube and are not the source of melanomas.[20]

Epidemiology

Uveal melanoma most often develops in the sixth decade of life. Although generally uncommon, it is the most common primary intraocular malignancy and the only primary intraocular disease in adults that can be fatal.[21] Death results from distant metastases. This tumor is rare in nonwhites whereas individuals with light-colored irises are at increased risk.[22,23] A slight preponderance in males was demonstrated.[22] The presence of uveal nevi (Color Plate XI) or ocular melanocytosis is thought to increase the risk of developing a uveal melanoma.

Although only around 10% of uveal melanoma cases seem to have a hereditable component,[24] mutations within the cell genome have been linked to this disease. Many investigators have reported karyotypic abnormalities in several different chromosomes. A striking feature in uveal melanomas was the association of anomalies in chromosomes 3 and 8 with ciliary body melanomas.[25,26] Specifically, a monosomy of chromosome 3 and additional copies of the long arm of chromosome 8 were frequent findings,[27] both of which were associated with a poor prognosis. The association of monosomy 3 with uveal melanoma was suggested to be a result of the deletion of a suppressor gene, whereas the abnormalities in chromosome 8 were thought to contribute to malignancy through an increase in gene dose of a promoter oncogene located on this chromosome.[28]

Clinical Features

Choroidal melanoma is characterized by an elevated, oval mass showing some intrinsic pigmentation, though nearly one-fourth of all melanomas are amelanotic. As the tumor grows, it can pierce through Bruch's membrane and appear as a mushroom-shaped (collar-button appearance) mass. This may be accompanied by the accumulation of yellow lipofuscin pigment in the retinal pigment epithelial cells. If large enough, it can result in secondary exudative detachment of the retina (Color Plate XII) and also possibly an area of the choroid.[29] Alternatively, choroidal melanomas can develop diffusely and involve a significant portion of the choroid (Color Plate XIII). Conditions most diagnostically similar to choroidal melanoma include retinal and choroidal detachment, metastatic tumor of the choroid, exudative age-related maculopathy, localized choroidal hemangioma, and a large choroidal nevus.[29] Transillumination is useful for differentiating pigmented choroidal melanomas from nonpigmented tumors, exudative retinal detachments, and choroidal detachments (Figure 6.2).

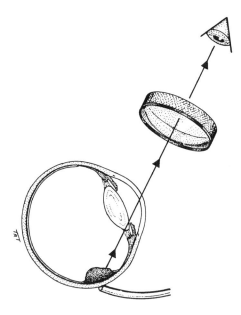

FIGURE 6.2.   Technique of scleral transillumination for the detection of pigmented choroidal melanoma. (Reprinted with permission from JJ Kanski. Clinical Ophthalmology [3rd ed]. London: Butterworth–Heinemann, 1994;214.)

Ciliary body melanomas can only be visualized when the pupil is dilated widely. In some cases, the presence of episcleral vessels draws the attention of the clinician to the possibility of such a tumor. Because it is difficult to spot in its early stages, ciliary body melanomas are often quite large at the time of diagnosis, particularly when a circumferential growth pattern is present. Large tumors can compress the lens equator and produce an astigmatic refractive error. Transillumination is effective in assessing tumor dimension and evaluating treatment strategies.[30] Two conditions that should be considered in the differential diagnosis of ciliary body melanomas are medulloepithelioma (malignant tumor derived from embryonic medullary canal) and leiomyoma (a benign smooth muscle tumor). However, these tumors are rare and generally occur in children and young women.

Iris melanomas usually present as a pigmented or nonpigmented nodule in the lower half of the iris.[30] These tumors are very slow growing, with reported cases showing no change for more than 30 years. They may be associated with spontaneous hyphema, localized lens opacities, distortion of the pupil, and ectropion uveae.[30] In nonpigmented tumors, an increased tumor vascularization can be seen. Conditions that can be initially mistaken for iris melanoma are large iris granulomas, leiomyomas, and iris nevi, the latter of which do not usually distort the pupil. For a summary of differential diagnoses for ocular melanomas, see Table 6.1.

TABLE 6.1
Differential Diagnoses for Ocular Melanoma

Choroidal melanoma
   Choroidal detachment
   Retinal detachment
   Metastatic tumor
   Exudative age-related maculopathy
   Localized choroidal hemangioma
   Large choroidal nevus
Ciliary body melanoma
   Medulloepithelioma
   Leiomyoma
Iris melanoma
   Granuloma
   Leiomyoma
   Nevus

Pathogenesis

As mentioned above, of the three types of uveal melanomas, choroidal and ciliary body melanomas are the most life threatening, causing death in about half of those afflicted. Death is not directly a result of the expansion of the primary tumor but rather of the growth of distant metastases, most commonly in the liver.[31] About 1% of patients with uveal melanoma simultaneously present with systemic metastases.[32]

Various factors contribute to metastatic potential and thus pathogenicity of uveal tumors. As expected, the larger the tumor the higher the mortality rate.[33] Results from the analysis of mortality based on tumor location have been equivocal. Hence, although several studies suggested that tumors that extended anterior to the eye's equator offered a poor prognosis, this may well have been due to the fact that such tumors were generally larger.[28,34,35] The morphologic features of the constituent cells within a uveal melanoma have also been linked to its metastatic potential. Three cell types have been described in such tumors, resulting in the following classification: spindle cell nevi, spindle cell melanoma, and mixed cell tumors.[36] More recently, the relative size of the tumor cell's nucleolar diameter was shown to be a more objective measure of patient survival, though the techniques used to obtain such information are difficult to perform, expensive, and time-consuming.[37,38]

The microcirculation patterns in choroidal and ciliary body melanomas have also been associated with metastatic potential. Although several vascular patterns were described for these tumors,[39] those displaying vascular loops, particularly when they form vascular networks composed of back-to-back closed loops, were associated with death from metastatic disease.[28,40] Interestingly, type VI collagen, which plays an important role in tissue and vascular remodeling,[41] was shown to be present in the microcirculation of choroidal and ciliary body melanomas.[42] Although type VI collagen is not present in the choroidal stroma and is present in only low levels in the choriocapillaris, it is produced by uveal melanomas,[42] which may facilitate the development of microvascular networks within these tumors, leading to an enhanced probability of tumor metastatic spread.

The metastatic potential of uveal melanomas is influenced not only by their ability to produce extracellular molecules such as collagen, but also by their ability to degrade molecules in the extracellular matrix. Human uveal melanoma cell lines were found to possess fibrinolytic activity, with the highest levels being present in tumors that had significant scleral invasion.[43] Furthermore, matrix metalloproteinases, enzymes involved in connective tissue remodeling, were also found in these cells.

Therapeutic Options

Iris melanomas should be monitored for growth every 6 months. The full extent of the lesion should be mapped by slit-lamp examination and gonioscopy.[30] In most cases involving small tumors in which growth has been detected, broad iridectomy is sufficient treatment. In the case of ciliary body melanomas, serial observation, charged particle radiation, localized radioactive plaques (brachytherapy), local resection, and enucleation are treatment options depending on the size and extent of the tumor. The use of charged particle radiation or localized radioactive plaques is referred to as *radiotherapy*. In certain cases it is more effective and patients have fewer complications than those undergoing surgical resection. Radioisotopes that have been used for radiotherapy include iodine 125, iridium 192, ruthenium 106, and radium 222, with cobalt 60 being reserved for the largest tumors.[30] Factors to consider in the treatment of choroidal melanomas include rate of tumor growth, size, location, and visual acuity. Large tumors require enucleation, though smaller tumors may be responsive to radiotherapy. Small tumors that do not touch the optic disc margin and are located at least 3 mm from the fovea are candidates for photocoagulation, but even in those meeting the criteria, many will still require follow-up enucleation.[30] In all cases where distant metastases have developed, systemic chemotherapy and immunotherapy are required, though the prognosis is poor in these patients.

Retinoblastoma

Retinoblastoma is a malignant ocular neoplasm of childhood that usually occurs before 3 years of age. Although it is the most common intraocular tumor of childhood, its incidence is only about 1 in 25,000 live births,[44] and

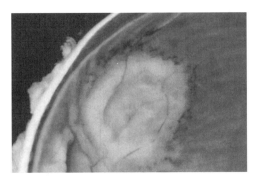

FIGURE 6.3.   Low-power photomicrograph of a retinoma in a patient who subsequently died from small cell carcinoma of the lung. More than 40 years earlier, this patient's fellow eye was enucleated because of retinoblastoma. (Reprinted with permission from WE Alberti, RH Sagerman. Radiotherapy of Intraocular and Orbital Tumors. New York: Springer, 1993;104.)

it accounts for only 1% of all childhood malignancies.[45] It arises within the nuclear layers of the retina from multiple foci in one or both eyes.[46] It has been estimated that approximately 1% of retinoblastomas spontaneously regress, implicating the immune system in retinal surveillance. Regression can occur in both unilateral and bilateral cases.[47] Regressed tumors are referred to as *retinomas* or *retinocytomas*, though these benign counterparts to retinoblastoma may have a different etiology. Retinomas are characterized by partial calcification and the presence of remnants of the tumor vasculature (Figure 6.3).[48] Other evidence of immune reactivity to retinoblastoma antigens includes the demonstration of in vitro cytotoxicity to a retinoblastoma cell line by immune cells derived from retinoblastoma patients and a positive DTH response to a crude tumor membrane extract.[49,50] Antigens reported to be expressed in retinoblastomas include rhodopsin and S antigen, which are present in normal photoreceptors, as well as the amacrine cell markers substance P and preproenkephalin.[51]

Epidemiology

It has been estimated that the incidence of retinoblastoma will increase over the next century. Reasons given include the increased environmental exposure to UV radiation as a result of ozone depletion and the enhanced survival into their reproductive years of children with familial retinoblastoma. Patients with familial retinoblastoma have a 50% risk of transmitting the disease to their progeny.

Retinoblastomas can arise as either a germinal or somatic mutation.[44] Multiple primary retinoblastomas, whether in one or both eyes, always result from a germinal mutation,[44] though many such cases present with

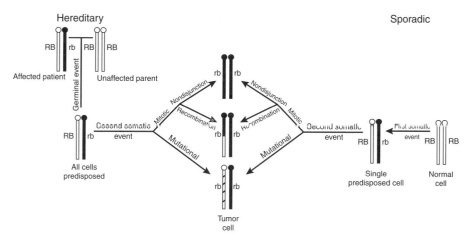

FIGURE 6.4. The two-hit hypothesis of retinoblastoma (RB,rb) formation. (Reprinted with permission from EL Schubert, MF Hansen, LC Strong. The retinoblastoma gene and its significance. Ann Med 1994;26:179–184.)

only one tumor.[52] The gene that has been implicated in hereditary retinoblastoma is called the *retinoblastoma gene*, or *RB1*, and it encodes for a protein that, in its unphosphorylated state, binds to DNA and prevents cell replication. It is located on the long arm of chromosome 13 and belongs to a class of genes called *tumor suppressors*,[53] which play an integral role in the control of the cell cycle. When an allele of the *RB1* gene is defective or missing, cells are predisposed to tumorigenesis by a second somatic event, perhaps induced by exposure to radiation or an environmental carcinogen. This second somatic event may take the form of mitotic nondisjunction, recombination, or mutation (Figure 6.4). In individuals who develop a nonhereditary form of retinoblastoma, somatic events must occur twice in the same cell. The notion that retinoblastoma (and tumors in general) results from two transforming events was formulated by Knudson and is called the *two-hit hypothesis*.[54,55]

In addition to retinoblastoma, a host of other human tumors have been shown to be associated with mutations in the *RB1* gene, including osteosarcoma, glioblastoma, and breast, lung, bladder, prostate, and ovarian cancer.[56] The incidence of osteogenic sarcomas and pineal or parasellar tumors in patients successfully treated for retinoblastoma is quite high. The association of these intracranial tumors with bilateral retinoblastoma is referred to as *trilateral retinoblastoma*.[44]

Clinical Features

The most common presenting feature of retinoblastoma is a white reflex in the pupil, called *leukocoria*, sometimes also referred to as the *cat's eye*

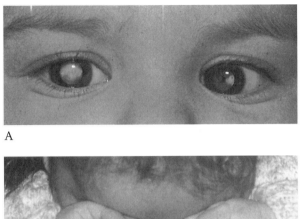

A

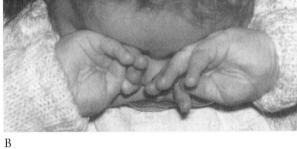

B

FIGURE 6.5. (A) Bilateral leukocoria in a 1-year-old child with gross bilateral ocular involvement. Note the convergent squint. (B) Affected children poke and rub their eyes, possibly to obtain some visual sensation by the production of phosphenes from manual stimulation. (Reprinted from DJ Spalton, RA Hitchings, PA Hunter. Atlas of Clinical Ophthalmology [2nd ed]. London: Wolfe, 1994;15.28. With permission from Mosby International, Inc.)

reflex (Figure 6.5). If the tumor originates in the macular region, a white reflex may be present even when the tumor is still relatively small. If it originates at the periphery of the retina, however, it can grow very large before presentation.[48] Other conditions that can present with leukocoria include *Toxocara* granuloma, caused by the nematode larva; anterior persistent hyperplastic primary vitreous; retinopathy of prematurity, and Coats' disease—though the latter is almost always unilateral and occurs later than retinoblastoma.[57] Additional presenting symptoms for retinoblastoma include strabismus and apparent intraocular inflammation and glaucoma, the latter resulting from either the tumor pushing the lens diaphragm forward or clogging the trabecular meshwork.[58] Poor vision is a presenting sign in only a minority of cases. In underdeveloped countries, advanced cases with extraocular extension are most often seen, and treatment is largely palliative.[44]

Retinoblastomas generally appear as pink masses protruding from the retina into the vitreous, usually showing areas of neovascularization on their surface.[48] Tumors can either grow from the inner surface of the retina into the vitreous, called *endophytic retinoblastomas*, or they may grow from the outer retinal surface toward the choroid, called *exophytic retinoblastomas*. Two characteristic features are a fluffy pattern of calcification and the seeding of tumor cells into the vitreous.[48] The latter sign, when accompanying a large tumor, bodes ill for patient survival. Tumors also characteristically produce high levels of lactate dehydrogenase, which enters the aqueous humor and can be measured to facilitate the differential diagnosis.

Pathogenesis

Retinoblastoma tumor cells are transformed photoreceptor cells. The cells may appear fully or partially differentiated. In the latter form, the cells take on the appearance of rosettes, referred to as *Flexner-Wintersteiner rosettes*, which usually appear in areas of undifferentiated malignant cells. Cells comprising the rosette share many features with fully differentiated photoreceptors, including tight junctions, cytoplasmic microtubules, cilia, and lamellated membranous structures resembling the disks of rod outer segments.[44] Tumors composed entirely of benign-appearing cells are considered to be retinocytomas.[44]

Extension of retinoblastoma growth outside the eye generally occurs an average of 6 months after its first symptoms.[59] Metastatic spread occurs along the optic nerve to the brain and subarachnoid space, hematogenously to the bones and viscera, and by lymphatics from extraocularly extended tumors. Extension of the tumor into the optic nerve, choroid, sclera, or orbit is associated with a poor prognosis.[60] In general, long-term survival rates are also low in patients with bilateral tumors.[30] The overall mortality rate for retinoblastoma is 15%.[30]

Treatment

The size and extent of the tumor are critical factors in assessing forms of treatment. Enucleation, taking a long stretch of optic nerve, is the most common treatment. Radiotherapy, using an external beam or iodine 125 or ruthenium 106 plaques, is used for small tumors. Photocoagulation with a xenon arc laser can also be used for small tumors confined to the retina. It has been suggested that photocoagulation should be applied around the tumor, rather than directly to it, so as to cut off its blood supply.[61] Lesions with a diameter less than 6 mm and a thickness less than 3 mm that are located at the ora serrata can be eradicated using transscleral cryotherapy.[62]

References

1. Cotran RS, Kumar V, Robbins SL (eds). Robbins' Pathologic Basis of Disease. Philadelphia: Saunders, 1994;273.

2. Niederkorn JY. The immunopathogenesis of ocular tumors. Prog Retin Eye Res 1995;14:505–526.

3. Ma D, Luyten GP, Luider TM, Niederkorn JY. Relationship between natural killer cell susceptibility and metastasis of human uveal melanoma cells in a murine model. Invest Ophthalmol Vis Sci 1995;36:435–441.

4. Apte R, Niederkorn JY. Isolation and characterization of a unique natural killer cell inhibitory factor present in the anterior chamber of the eye. J Immunol 1996;156:2667–2673.

5. Niederkorn JY. Immunoregulation of intraocular tumors. Eye 1997;11:249–254.

6. Meecham WJ, Char DH, Kaleta-Michaels S. Infiltrating lymphocytes and antigen expression in uveal melanoma. Ophthalmic Res 1992;24:20–26.

7. Ksander BR, Rubsamen PE, Olsen KR, et al. Studies of tumor-infiltrating lymphocytes from a human choroidal melanoma. Invest Ophthalmol Vis Sci 1991;32:3198–3208.

8. Knisely TL, Luckenbach MW, Fischer BJ, Niederkorn JY. Destructive and nondestructive patterns of immune rejection of syngeneic intraocular tumors. J Immunol 1987;138:4515–4523.

9. Knisely TL, Niederkorn JY. Immunologic evaluation of spontaneous regression of an intraocular murine melanoma. Invest Ophthalmol Vis Sci 1990; 31:247–257.

10. Ma D, Comerford S, Bellingham D, et al. Capacity of simian virus 40 T antigen to induce self-tolerance but not immunological privilege in the anterior chamber of the eye. Transplantation 1994;57:718–725.

11. Jiang LQ, Jorquera M, Streilein JW. Subretinal space and vitreous cavity as immunologically privileged sites for retinal allografts. Invest Ophthalmol Vis Sci 1993;34:3347–3354.

12. Durie FH, Campbell AM, Lee WR, Damato BE. Analysis of lymphocytic infiltration in uveal melanoma. Invest Ophthalmol Vis Sci 1990;31: 2106–2110.

13. Knisely TL, Niederkorn JY. Emergence of a dominant cytotoxic T lymphocyte (CTL) antitumor effector from tumor infiltrating cells in the anterior chamber of the eye. Cancer Immunol Immunother 1990;30:323–330.

14. Ma D, Alizadeh H, Comerford SA, et al. Rejection of intraocular tumors from transgenic mice by tumor-infiltrating lymphocytes. Curr Eye Res 1994; 13:361–369.

15. Mulcahy KA, Rimoldi D, Brasseur F, et al. Infrequent expression of the MAGE gene family in uveal melanomas. Int J Cancer 1996;66:738–742.

16. Davidorf FH, Lang JR. Immunology and Immunotherapy of Malignant Uveal Melanomas. In GA Peyman, DJ Apple, DR Sanders (eds), Intraocular Tumors. New York: Appleton-Century-Crofts, 1977;119–133.

17. Kremer I, Gilad E, Kahan E, et al. Necrosis and lymphocytic infiltration in choroidal melanomas. Acta Ophthalmol Scand 1991;69:347–351.

18. Whelchel JC, Farah SE, McLean IW, Burnier MN. Immunochemistry of infiltrating lymphocytes in uveal malignant melanoma. Invest Ophthalmol Vis Sci 1993;34:2603–2606.

19. Ksander BR, Bando Y, Acevedo J, Streilein JW. Infiltration and accumulation of precursor cytotoxic T cells increase with time in progressively growing ocular tumors. Cancer Res 1991;51:3153–3158.

20. Garner A, McCartney A. Immunology of Ocular Tumors. In S Lightman (ed), Immunology of Eye Diseases. Lancaster, UK: Kluwer, 1989;131.

21. Egan KM, Seddon JM, Glynn RJ, et al. Epidemiologic aspects of uveal melanoma. Surv Ophthalmol 1988;32:239–251.

22. Shammas HF, Blodi FC. Prognostic factors in choroidal and ciliary body melanomas. Arch Ophthalmol 1977;95:63–69.

23. Tucker MA, Shields JA, Hartge P, et al. Sunlight exposure as risk factor for intraocular malignant melanoma. N Engl J Med 1985;313:789–792.

24. Greene MH, Fraumeni J. The Hereditary Variant of Malignant Melanoma. In WH Clark, LI Goldman, MJ Mastrangelo (eds), Human Malignant Melanoma. New York: Grune & Stratton, 1979;139–166.

25. Sisley K, Cottam D, Rennie IG, et al. Cytogenetics of uveal melanoma. Invest Ophthalmol Vis Sci 1992;33(suppl):1243.

26. Prescher G, Bornfeld N, Horsthemke B, Becher R. Chromosomal aberrations defining uveal melanoma of poor prognosis. Lancet 1992;339:691–692.

27. Sisley K, Rennie IG, Parsons MA, et al. Abnormalities of chromosomes 3 and 8 in posterior uveal melanoma correlate with prognosis. Genes Chromosomes Cancer 1997;19:22–28.

28. Rennie IG. The Ashton lecture. Uveal melanoma: the past, the present and the future. Eye 1997;11:255–264.

29. Char DH (ed). Clinical Ocular Oncology (2nd ed). Philadelphia: Lippincott–Raven, 1997;189.

30. Kanski JJ (ed). Clinical Ophthalmology (3rd ed). London: Butterworth–Heinemann, 1994;207–221.

31. Char DH. Metastatic choroidal melanoma. Am J Ophthalmol 1978;86:76–80.

32. Char DH (ed). Clinical Ocular Oncology (2nd ed). Philadelphia: Lippincott–Raven, 1997;115.

33. Diener-West M, Hawkins BS, Markowitz JA, Schachat AP. A review of mortality from choroidal melanoma. II. A meta-analysis of 5-year mortality rates following enucleation, 1966 through 1988. Arch Ophthalmol 1992;110: 245–250.

34. Seddon JM, Albert DM, Lavin PT, Robinson N. A prognostic factor study of disease-free interval and survival following enucleation for uveal melanoma. Arch Ophthalmol 1983;101:1894–1899.

35. McLean MJ, Foster WD, Zimmerman LE. Prognostic factors in small malignant melanomas of choroid and ciliary body. Arch Ophthalmol 1977;95:48–58.

36. McLean IW, Foster WD, Zimmerman LE, Gamel JW. Modifications of Callender's classification of uveal melanoma of the Armed Forces Institute of Pathology. Am J Ophthalmol 1983;96:502–509.

37. Gamel JW, McLean I, Greenberg RA, et al. Objective assessment of the malignant potential of intraocular melanomas with standard microslides stained with hematoxylin-eosin. Hum Pathol 1985;16:689–692.

38. Donoso LA, Augsburger JJ, Shields JA, et al. Metastatic uveal melanoma. Correlation between survival time and cytomorphometry of primary tumors. Arch Ophthalmol 1986;104:76–78.

39. Folberg R, Mehaffey M, Gardner LM, et al. The microcirculation of choroidal and ciliary body melanomas. Eye 1997;11:227–238.

40. Rummelt V, Folberg R, Woolson RF, et al. Relation between the microcirculation architecture and the aggressive behavior of ciliary body melanomas. Ophthalmology 1995;102:844–851.

41. Sage EH, Vernon RB. Regulation of angiogenesis by extracellular matrix: the growth and the glue. J Hypertens 1994;12(suppl):S145–S152.

42. Daniels KJ, Boldt HC, Martin JA, et al. Expression of type VI collagen in uveal melanoma: role in pattern formation and tumor progression. Lab Invest 1996;75:55–66.

43. Cottam DW, Rennie IG, Woods K, et al. Gelatinolytic metalloproteinase secretion patterns in ocular melanoma. Invest Ophthalmol Vis Sci 1992;33: 1923–1927.

44. McLean IW. Retinoblastomas, Retinocytomas, and Pseudoretinoblastomas. In WH Spencer (ed), Ophthalmic Pathology. Philadelphia: Saunders, 1996;1332.

45. Alberti WE, Sagerman RH. Diagnosis and Management of Retinoblastoma. In WE Alberti, RH Sagerman (eds), Radiotherapy of Intraocular and Orbital Tumors. Berlin: Springer, 1993;101.

46. Friedlander MH. Allergy and Immunology of the Eye. New York: Raven Press, 1993;321.

47. Khodadoust AA, Roozitalab HM, Smith RE, Green WR. Spontaneous regression of retinoblastoma. Surv Ophthalmol 1977;21:467–478.

48. Ellsworth RM, Boxrad CA. Retinoblastoma. In Duane's Ophthalmology on CD-ROM. Philadelphia: Lippincott–Raven, 1996.

49. Char DH, Ellsworth R, Rabson AS, et al. Cell-mediated immunity to a retinoblastoma tissue culture line in patients with retinoblastoma. Am J Ophthalmol 1974;78:5–11.

50. Char DH, Herberman RB. Cutaneous delayed hypersensitivity responses of patients with retinoblastoma to standard recall antigens and crude membrane extracts of retinoblastoma tissue culture cells. Am J Ophthalmol 1974;78: 40–44.

51. Garner A, McCartney A. Immunology of Ocular Tumors. In S Lightman (ed), Immunology of Eye Diseases. Lancaster, UK: Kluwer, 1989;136.

52. Yandell DW, Poremba C. Genetics of retinoblastoma: implications for other human cancers. Med Pediatr Oncol 1996;1(suppl):25–28.

53. Whyte P. The retinoblastoma protein and its relatives. Semin Cancer Biol 1995;6:83–90.

54. Knudson AG Jr. Mutation and cancer: statistical study of retinoblastoma. Proc Natl Acad Sci U S A 1971;68:820–823.

55. Knudson AG Jr. Hereditary cancers disclose a class of cancer genes. Cancer 1989;63:1888–1891.

56. Schubert EL, Hansen MF, Strong LC. The retinoblastoma gene and its significance. Ann Med 1994;26:177–184.

57. Lean IW. Retinoblastomas, Retinocytomas, and Pseudoretinoblastomas. In WH Spencer (ed), Ophthalmic Pathology. Philadelphia: Saunders, 1996;1376.

58. Pavan-Langston D. Manual of Ocular Diagnosis and Therapy (4th ed). Boston: Little, Brown, 1996;292.

59. Erwenne CM, Franco EL. Age and lateness of referral as determinants of extra-ocular retinoblastoma. Ophthalmic Paediatr Genet 1989;10:179–184.

60. Kopelman JE, McLean IW, Rosenberg SH. Multivariate analysis of risk factors for metastasis in retinoblastoma treated by enucleation. Ophthalmology 1987;94:371–377.

61. Shields JA, Shields CL, Donoso LA, Lieb W. Current treatment of retinoblastoma. Trans Penn Acad Ophthalmol Otolaryngol 1989;41:818–822.

62. Alberti WE, Sagerman RH. Diagnosis and Management of Retinoblastoma. In WE Alberti, RH Sagerman (eds), Radiotherapy of Intraocular and Orbital Tumors. Berlin: Springer, 1993;107.

CHAPTER 7

Corneal Transplantation

From an optical point of view, I also had no better results with my operations [than did Fuchs and von Hippel], until a case at the end of this past year had a surprisingly favorable result. At present, after almost seven months, the transparency of the transplanted lobe [cornea] is preserved intact, visual acuity has remained unchanged at the same level for an extended period of time, so that it seems justifiable for me to report the details of the case more specifically.*

Clinicians have aspired for more than a century to successfully transplant the cornea into individuals suffering from irreversible corneal opacification. This chapter explores various aspects of corneal transplantation, including indications for the procedure, the clinical criteria for graft rejection and its risk factors, pharmacologic approaches for the prevention and reversal of rejection, risks of disease transmission from donor to recipient, and xenoengraftment. The anatomy and immunobiology of the cornea are reviewed as a prelude to these discussions.

Anatomy of the Cornea

The transparent cornea constitutes the anterior sixth of the outer wall of the eye. It has an anterior radius of curvature of about 7.7 mm compared with a 13.5 mm curvature for the sclera, which accounts for its protrusion from the surface of the eyeball.[1] Corneal thickness varies from 500 mm at its center to 100 mm peripherally, resulting in a difference in curvature between the anterior and posterior surfaces. The cornea consists of an epithelial layer that is approximately five cell layers, or 50 mm, thick. The apical cells exhibit a glycocalyx that attaches loosely to the mucous layer of the tear film and also binds to immunoglobulin molecules in the aqueous tear film layer.[1,2]

---

*From the description of the first reported successful corneal allograft by Eduard Zirm entitled "A successful total keratoplasty," published in 1906 (translated from the German by Esther Griswold).

Lying immediately beneath the epithelial cells of primate eyes is Bowman's membrane, a 30-mm thick acellular layer containing various collagen types. It merges anteriorly with the lamina densa of the epithelial basal lamina and its collagen fibrils become continuous posteriorly with the underlying stroma. Indications are that Bowman's layer contributes to the strength and stiffness of the cornea and may play a role in the restoration of corneal shape following keratorefractive surgery.[3] Beneath Bowman's layer is the corneal stroma, a 450-mm thick fibrous tissue layer composed predominantly of type I collagen, the fibrils of which have a relatively uniform diameter and are arranged in a highly ordered fashion. It is thought that light scatter induced by each fibril is canceled by the scatter caused by adjacent fibrils, thus contributing to corneal transparency.[4] Other factors thought to be responsible for corneal transparency are the stromal glycosaminoglycans, which play a role in maintaining collagen interfibrillar spacing, and the cornea's lack of blood and lymphatic vessels.[5]

The final two layers of the cornea are Descemet's membrane (the basal lamina of the endothelium) and the endothelium. Descemet's membrane is about 10 mm thick and tends to coil inward when incised or ruptured, a feature that allows it to accommodate reversible corneal swelling. It also plays a role in evenly distributing tension and in preventing gross deformities of the tissue.[6] Both Bowman's layer and Descemet's membrane play a role in preventing the spread of infection; unlike Bowman's layer, however, Descemet's membrane can be regenerated after injury.[7]

The single layer of endothelial cells belies its important role in maintaining normal corneal deturgescence and transparency. Tight junctions between neighboring cells prevent appreciable movement of aqueous humor into the cornea; fluid that does leak past these cells is counterbalanced by the active transport of fluid by the endothelial cells.[1] When the endothelial cells are damaged or their numbers reduced, such transport may fail to keep pace with fluid diffusion, resulting in the development of stromal edema. More often than not it is the endothelial cell that is the target of immune attack in corneal graft rejection. The endothelial cells also play a role in the diffusion of nutrients from the aqueous humor to the avascular cornea.

The corneal epithelium is innervated by both sensory and sympathetic nerves. There is also some sensory innervation of the stroma but no innervation to Descemet's membrane or the endothelium. Release of neuropeptides from sensory corneal nerves contributes to the immune privilege of the cornea and anterior chamber.[8]

Immunology of the Cornea

The deceptively simple structure of the cornea belies its important role not only in providing an intact refractive surface but also in regulating the ocular immune response. As described in more detail in Chapter 2, the cornea exhibits various features that afford it a privileged immune status. Specifically, the corneal stroma lacks a vascular supply and a lymphatic drainage, and the central cornea (unlike the limbus) lacks antigen-presenting cells (i.e., Langerhans' cells). In addition, the different layers of the cornea have been shown to produce immunosuppressive factors.[8] Explants of corneal tissue from BALB/c mice were shown to have the ability to suppress T cell activation in a mixed lymphocyte reaction (MLR). Although the cytokine transforming growth factor–beta (TGF-β) is known to be secreted by iris and ciliary body cells into the aqueous humor and to be responsible for the suppression of certain intraocular immunologic reactions such as delayed-type hypersensitivity (DTH), only a small amount of TGF-β is produced by the cornea, specifically by corneal endothelial cells.[9] Furthermore, it was shown using blocking antibodies to TGF-β that the immunosuppressive factor produced by the cornea was not TGF-β.[10] Human corneal stromal fibroblasts produce a factor capable of inhibiting the allogeneic MLR.[11] Interferon-gamma (IFN-γ), normally an immune-stimulating cytokine, intensified the inhibitory effect of these cells though indomethacin, a prostaglandin inhibitor, had no effect, suggesting that the suppressive factor was not prostaglandin. Interestingly, the immunosuppressive effect of a soluble factor released from epithelial cells derived from human corneo-scleral-conjunctival rims was inhibited by indomethacin.[12]

Although corneal tissues have been shown to be immunosuppressive, they also secrete a multitude of cytokines and other immune-activating factors. Specifically, corneal epithelial cells secrete interleukin-1 (IL-1), IL-6, IL-8, tumor necrosis factor–alpha (TNF-α), IFN-γ, complement protein C5a, and prostaglandins.[13] Fibroblasts in the stroma (i.e., keratocytes) secrete IL-1, IL-6, IL-8, and TNF-α.[13-15] Corneal endothelial cells may also secrete IL-8[16] and constitutively express the adhesion molecules, intercellular adhesion molecule–1 (ICAM-1, the principal ligand responsible for leukocyte binding during inflammation) and CD44, which play a role in lymphocyte binding to, and entrapment by, high endothelial venules.[17,18] In addition to cytokines, antigen-presenting Langerhans' cells have been described in the cornea[19]; nearly all of these have been located in the corneal limbus with only a few scattered cells present in the central cornea.[20] Corticosteroids and TGF-β have been shown to inhibit the migration of Langerhans' cells into the central cornea, whereas cytokines such as IL-1, TNF-α, and others promote central corneal Langerhans' cells chemotaxis.[21,22] Langerhans' cells can migrate into the central cornea in response to infectious agents,[21] chemical irritants,[23] or localized damage.[24] The presence of Langerhans' cells in the central cornea can, as is discussed later, abrogate anterior chamber–associated immune deviation (ACAID) and promote corneal allograft rejection. Finally, corneal epithelial cells express class II histocompatibility antigens and stimulate an immune response after IFN-γ treatment.[25]

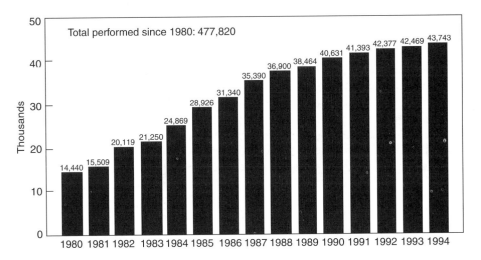

FIGURE 7.1.   Annual frequency of penetrating keratoplasties. (Reprinted with permission from the Eye Bank Association of America, Washington, D.C.)

Corneal Transplantation

According to the Eye Bank Association of America, approximately 40,000 corneal transplantations, also called *penetrating keratoplasties*, are performed each year in the United States and Canada (Figure 7.1). Not surprisingly, based on the accessibility of the tissue and its immune-privileged status, the success of this procedure is nearly unparalleled in the field of tissue and organ transplantation.[26] Graft failure can occur as a result of technical problems, infection, or graft rejection. This chapter starts with a discussion of the indications for performing a corneal transplantation and preoperative and postoperative care. The major focus, however, is an analysis of the mechanism and factors influencing graft rejection and a discussion of treatments to prevent and reverse rejection. The chapter concludes with a discussion of the possibility of transmission of donor diseases through corneal transplantation and a brief word about corneal xenografts.

Indications

The indications for performing a penetrating keratoplasty are diverse, but most fall into three categories: optical, tectonic, and therapeutic.[27] A patient with a cornea that is opaque or distorted significantly as a result of astigmatism is a candidate for a transplant for optical reasons. A tectonic penetrating keratoplasty, also called a *reconstructive penetrating kerato-plasty*, is performed to restore the integrity of the globe following perforation. Therapeutic keratoplasty is performed when the cornea is diseased as a result of an infection that has not responded to medications such as antibiotics or as a result of previous eye surgery. The latter case is arguably the most common indication for this surgery. Specifically, corneal engraftment is performed to replace an edematous cornea that results from either an aphakic or pseudophakic lensectomy (i.e., cataract surgery to remove or replace a cloudy lens, respectively). In a procedure called the *triple procedure,* removal of an opacified lens together with its replacement with a lens implant is performed in combination with a penetrating keratoplasty.[28] This is usually performed in older patients for whom the rapid attainment of enhanced visual acuity is paramount, even at the expense of increased optical risk.[28]

Preoperative and Postoperative Care

A thorough ocular history and examination, including the performance of visual acuity testing, are necessary prerequisites to surgery. Abnormalities of any kind in the production of the tear film are a contraindication for surgery. Increased intraocular pressure before surgery bodes ill for postoperative prognosis. The proper diagnosis of the ocular pathology that necessitated the surgery is required because it has a bearing on surgical approach. Various preoperative medications are usually given to maximize the chance of successful engraftment including the prophylactic use of topical antibiotics or 2% pilocarpine in phakic patients to induce miosis and protect the lens.[27]

Topical agents are applied postoperatively to prevent rejection and infection.[27] These include prednisolone sodium phosphate, acetate, neomycin, and polymyxin. Patients at high risk for viral reactivation such as those receiving a graft as a result of corneal opacity due to viral keratitis can receive antiviral agents such as oral acyclovir. Sutures are usually removed between 2 and 3 months after surgery. The most common factor that limits visual acuity after surgery is astigmatism.[27] This can result in spite of surgical and postsurgical efforts to limit refractive error.

Although graft failure can occur for a host of reasons, the most common cause in patients with initially successful engraftment is graft rejection.

Graft Rejection

Clinical Criteria for Graft Rejection

Several clinical criteria are used to define graft rejection, as outlined by Thiel[29] (Table 7.1). Rejection generally appears after 3 weeks and is confined primarily to the graft. In nearly all cases and regardless of the corneal layer affected, rejection begins at the graft margin and progresses across the entire graft. Perhaps the most common type of corneal rejection involves the endothelium and is foreshadowed by stromal edema accompanied by vessel ingrowth into the stroma and the accumulation of inflammatory cells on the endothelium (i.e., keratic precipitates) (Color Plate XIV). There

TABLE 7.1
Clinical Criteria for Graft Rejection

Process generally begins after 3 wks
Inflammation is confined primarily to graft
Rejection begins at graft margin but can spread over entire graft
In mild reactions, endothelial reaction line is usually recognizable

---

may be a visible line at the boundary between the graft and host tissue called a *Khodadoust line,* representing the collection of leukocytes that ultimately advances over the entire surface of the cornea, leaving ravaged corneal tissue in its wake.[30] Corneal endothelial destruction can occur in as rapidly as 2 days, resulting in an edematous graft and a marked loss of vision.[29] Graft rejection can also begin as epithelial rejection (Color Plate XV), characterized by a red eye, reduced visual acuity, increased lacrimation, and foreign body sensation.

The fact that corneal rejection occurs presupposes the presence of immunogenic antigens in the graft. During the afferent limb of the rejection response, these antigens activate recipient immune cells. How this is accomplished depends on the nature of the triggering antigen. Although it seems reasonable to suggest that histocompatibility (MHC) antigens in the graft would play a role in this regard, the data, as discussed below, are not clear-cut. Various immune effectors have been implicated in the efferent limb of the corneal rejection response. Activated T cells were isolated from rejected corneas, with both helper CD4+ and cytotoxic CD8+ cells being represented.[31] Although CD4+ cells are the dominant subset at the initiation of rejection, their numbers decline thereafter as the number of CD8+ cytotoxic cells increase.[32,33] Depletion of both of these subsets with monoclonal antibodies significantly reduces the incidence of rejection, as does depletion of CD4+ cells alone, but depletion of CD8+ cells alone is without effect.[34,35] Although cytotoxic T cells were shown to target donor antigens,[36] the prevailing view is that CD4+ cells play the more important role in rejection directly, indirectly, or both through their release of cytokines.

Various cytokines have been implicated in corneal graft rejection. Elevated levels of macrophage migration inhibition factor, a cytokine known to be present in human corneal epithelial and endothelial cells,[37] were found in the aqueous humor of rabbits during the active phase of rejection.[38] TNF-α has been implicated as a rejection marker since high levels were found before graft rejection.[39] Polymerase chain reaction analysis of corneal tissue during experimental corneal transplantation revealed increased IL-6 expression after postoperative day 12, maximal IL-2 and IFN-γ expression on day 12, and an increased expression of TNF-α beginning on day 7.[39] Messenger RNA (mRNA) expression did not always correlate with secretion; for example, corneal grafts did not produce IL-6.[40] Not only has IL-2 been shown to be elevated during graft rejection[39,41] but antagonists of IL-2 receptor binding also suppressed corneal rejection.[42,43]

The role of adhesion molecules on corneal stromal and endothelial cells in graft rejection has also been investigated. The binding of these ligands to receptors on immune cells is known to facilitate inflammation in various tissues. In one study involving seven penetrating keratoplasty specimens with graft failure, six were found to express ICAM-1 on keratocytes and endothelial cells.[44] The level of expression positively correlated with the severity of inflammation. Lymphocyte function–associated antigen-1 (LFA-1), the receptor for ICAM-1, was found on the surface of leukocytes aggregating in the areas of increased expression of ICAM-1. TNF-α was shown to regulate the expression of ICAM-1.[45] Anti–LFA-1 antibody treatment significantly reduced the incidence of orthotopic corneal graft rejection, though it was ineffective in preimmunized hosts.[46,47] Very late antigen-4 (VLA-4), a receptor for vascular cellular adhesion molecule-1, has been implicated in allograft rejection and administration of a monoclonal antibody to VLA-4 in mice suppressed acute corneal allograft rejection.[48]

Evidence of a role for anticorneal antibodies in graft rejection has been limited.[49] Although recipient animals displayed an antigraft antibody response, it peaked about a week after graft rejection and was weaker than that which developed following skin grafting. Neither the presence of antibodies before corneal transplantation nor their appearance after engraftment had a predictive value for corneal graft survival.[50]

Risk Factors for Rejection

Genetic.   The obvious candidate genes that might play a role in corneal graft rejection are those of the MHC. Recall from Chapter 1 that MHC class I antigens are present on most body cells whereas class II antigens are restricted to cells of the immune system. In all other transplantation models, the general belief has been that the more alike donor and recipient MHC genes were, the more likely it was that the donor organ would be accepted. The data in corneal transplantation, however, have not been clear-cut, with some studies suggesting that HLA class I matching facilitates graft acceptance,[51,52] and others, most notably the U.S. multicenter collaborative study called the Collaborative Corneal Transplantation Studies (CCTS), concluded that matching of HLA-A,B (class I) or HLA-DR (class II) antigens has no effect on overall graft survival, the incidence of irreversible rejection, or the incidence of rejection episodes.[53]

The equivocal role of MHC antigens in corneal transplantation led to the investigation of other potentially more consequential genetic markers. These included minor histocompatibility (H) antigens and ABO antigens. High-risk grafts disparate for minor H antigens were shown to be rejected more frequently than were MHC class I or II disparate grafts.[54,55] In most

TABLE 7.2
Effects of Antigen Cross-Matching on Corneal Allograft Survival

Antigens	*Effect of Donor/Recipient Match on Allograft Survival*
MHC class I (HLA-A,B)	None
MHC class II (HLA-DR)	None
ABO	Beneficial
Minor H antigens	Beneficial

organ grafts, it is believed that donor-derived class II+ passenger leukocytes in the graft play a role in stimulating rejection by directly presenting foreign antigens to recipient T cells (i.e., by the "direct pathway" outlined in Chapter 1). Because nonvascularized donor corneas are deficient in such cells (e.g., Langerhans' cells), host reactivity to graft antigens is thought to occur "indirectly" by presentation of donor antigens by recipient Langerhans' cells to recipient T cells. Because normal corneal grafts have reduced levels of class I and II antigens, it was theorized that minor H antigens show reduced competition for presentation to the host and thus their significance as transplantation antigens is amplified.[55]

ABO-compatible grafts were shown to have been rejected at nearly half the rate of ABO-incompatible grafts in the high-risk cases studied in the CCTS. In low-risk transplants, there was no difference between these two groups.[56] The beneficial role of ABO matching in corneal transplantation mirrors the results obtained in several other transplantation studies involving other organs. These results are summarized in Table 7.2.

Immunologic

Role of Neovascularization and Langerhans' cells.   As mentioned, the cornea is an immunologically privileged site because it lacks blood/lymphatic vessels and antigen-presenting Langerhans' cells in the central cornea, and as a result of ACAID that is mediated by the release of factors by the cornea, ciliary body, and iris. Neovascularization of the recipient cornea has been associated with a significantly increased risk of rejection. Evidence in animal models in which neovascularization of the central cornea was induced by suturing[8] showed a migration of Langerhans' cells into the cornea with an accompanying loss of the ability of these eyes to support ACAID. Induction of Langerhans' cells migration has also been demonstrated by chemical stimulation with dinitrofluorobenzene[57] and by the instillation of either sterile latex beads or formalin-killed *Staphylococcus aureus*.[21] In the latter case, migration of Langerhans' cells was thought to be influenced by corneal epithelial cell release of IL-1 after phagocytosis.

The growth of new blood, and possibly lymphatic, vessels into a graft facilitates both the afferent and efferent limbs of the immune response to corneal tissue antigens. As mentioned above, data suggest that minor H antigens, which are processed by indirect presentation, may be more important than MHC antigens in corneal graft rejection. The induced migration of recipient Langerhans' cells by neovascularization facilitates this form of activation.

Certainly, experience has taught that neovascularization of graft beds resulting from injury or disease, an increased presence of Langerhans' cells in the graft, or both, in human corneal transplantation is associated with increased risk of rejection. For example, the prognosis in patients suffering from a herpes simplex virus (HSV) infection or keratitis, in which nearly 500 Langerhans' cells are observed per mm^2 of corneal tissue is poor; patients with keratoconus, who display between 0 and 25 Langerhans' cells per mm^2, have an excellent prognosis.[58] Topical angiostatic agents have restored corneal immune privilege,[59] and strategies to decrease corneal Langerhans' cells, such as by UV-B radiation,[60] improved corneal graft survival.

Role of Anterior Chamber–Associated Immune Deviation.   Recall that ACAID is characterized by the systemic inhibition of DTH and complement-fixing antibody formation in response to antigens in the aqueous humor. ACAID induced by alloantigens in corneal grafts has been speculated to be one of the reasons why these grafts show relative protection from rejection. Mice bearing long-term corneal allografts demonstrated suppression of alloantigen-specific DTH, whereas animals that rejected their grafts developed normal DTH to donor alloantigens.[61] ACAID was lost following corneal neovascularization induced by suturing of the central cornea[8] and following Langerhans' cells migration into the central cornea.[62] However, the induction of donor-specific ACAID before surgery effectively prolonged corneal allograft survival even in "high-risk" eyes in which the cornea was engrafted onto a vascularized bed.[63] Successful ACAID induction thus appears critical for successful corneal transplantation.

ACAID can be induced directly by the injection of antigens into the anterior chamber. When donor-derived, B cell–enriched immune cells were injected into the anterior chamber of recipient rats, the success rate of corneal allografts increased by 65%.[64,65] This finding was also seen in preimmune hosts injected intraocularly with whole irradiated donor spleen cells,[66] class II negative donor spleen cells,[67] or corneal endothelial cells.[68] When central corneal fragments were placed into the anterior chamber, ACAID was induced but its onset was delayed. The delay was speculated to be dictated by persistence of donor epithelial cells on the graft that promote DTH. Once the epithelium was lost, DTH disappeared and ACAID emerged.[69]

Pharmacologic Approaches to Prevent or Reverse Rejection

For most low-risk patients, postoperative immunosuppression consists of topical corticosteroid drops; one cocktail in use is 1.0% prednisolone and 0.1% dexamethasone, tapered over a prolonged period. In some cases, a subconjunctival corticosteroid injection is given at the completion of surgery.[68] Extra vigilance is exercised in high-risk patients, for example, patients with a vascularized graft bed, previous graft failure, or a predisposing corneal disease. In these patients, nighttime use of a steroid ointment is often used. Antiviral and antibacterial agents are sometimes also used in corneal transplant recipients, depending on the underlying risk factors for graft failure.

Cyclosporin and FK506, perhaps the most widely used immunosuppressive agents for the prevention and treatment of solid organ rejection, have been examined for their efficacy in corneal transplantation. Although one study failed to show any beneficial effect of systemic cyclosporin,[70] most others demonstrated its effectiveness in preventing human corneal allograft rejection.[71–73] The beneficial effects of the drug seemed to linger following treatment. The high cost of cyclosporin combined with its documented negative side effects preclude its generalized use for the prevention of corneal graft rejection. These concerns prompted investigations into its potential topical use. When applied to the surface of the eye, it reaches a high concentration in all layers of the cornea but remains fairly low in aqueous humor.[74] Application of the drug through collagen shields raised its concentration in aqueous humor. Although some have shown a beneficial effect of topical cyclosporin in preventing corneal graft rejection,[75,76] others have not.[68] Thus, the parameters for successful use of this drug in humans must await further investigation.

As with cyclosporin, systemic administration of FK506 prolonged corneal graft survival in animals.[77] Topical administration of FK506 to rabbits[78] and rats[79] prevented allograft rejection. It was also found to prolong xenograft survival in the rat keratoplasty model.[80]

Transmission of Donor Disease through Corneal Transplants

Transmission of donor-derived diseases is always a concern when transplanting tissues or organs because they can be serious or even life threatening. Diseases that have been transmitted by corneas include rabies, Creutzfeldt-Jakob disease, cytomegalovirus, HSV, and hepatitis B. Bacterial and fungal contaminants have also been passed to recipients.[81] To date, no case of human immunodeficiency virus transmission resulted from the inadvertent transplantation of corneas from seropositive donors.[82] Even though transmission of hepatitis B was reported from two donors,[83] it has been argued that the current eye-banking standards appear to be appropriately protective of the health of cornea recipients.[84]

Corneal Xenografts

If corneas from other species could be successfully transplanted into humans, the shortage of donor corneas would be alleviated. In fact, such an approach was attempted nearly 160 years ago. A major barrier hindering the use of solid organ xenografts is hyperacute graft rejection mediated by the recipient's preexisting, complement-fixing antibodies directed against the graft's endothelium. These antibodies rapidly promote intravascular thrombosis. The fact that the cornea is not vascularized has fueled the hopes of investigators that discordant corneal xenografts would not be hyperacutely rejected. Even though classic hyperacute rejection does not occur in xenografted corneas,[85] corneal xenografts do undergo accelerated damage that is mediated by a preexisting antibody.[86] The primary cause of xenograft failure appears to be corneal endothelial injury mediated by antibody attack.[87] This humoral response is followed in a week or two by a cell-mediated response that causes further destruction. The presence of a humoral immune component in xenograft rejection differentiates it from allograft rejection, which is primarily a cell-mediated response. Interestingly, cyclosporin effectively retarded the growth of new vessels in corneal xenografts and prolonged their survival.[80]

References

1. Smolek MK, Klyce SD. Foundation Cornea. In W Tasman, EA Jaeger (eds), Duane's Ophthalmology on CD-ROM. Philadelphia: Lippincott–Raven Publishers, 1997.
2. Gipson IK, Yankauckas M, Spurr-Michaud SJ, et al. Characteristics of a glycoprotein in the ocular surface glycocalyx. Invest Ophthalmol Vis Sci 1992; 33:218–227.
3. Hanna KD, Jouve FE, Waring GO III. Preliminary computer simulation of the effects of radial keratotomy. Arch Ophthalmol 1989;107:911–918.
4. Maurice DM. The structure and transparency of the cornea. J Physiol 1957; 136:263–286.
5. Cintron C, Covington HI. Proteoglycan distribution in developing rabbit cornea. J Histochem Cytochem 1990;38:675–684.
6. Kuwabara T. The Eye. In L Weiss (ed), Cell and Tissue Biology. Baltimore: Urban & Schwarzenberg, 1988;1078.
7. Ross MH, Reith EJ, Romrell LJ. Histology: A Text and Atlas. Norwalk, CT: Williams & Wilkins, 1989;716.
8. Streilein JW, Bradley D, Sano Y, Sonoda Y. Immunosuppressive properties of tissues obtained from eyes with experimentally manipulated corneas. Invest Ophthalmol Vis Sci 1996;37:413–424.
9. Wilson SE, Lloyd SA. Epidermal growth factor and its receptor, basic fibroblast growth factor, transforming growth factor beta-1, and interleukin-1a

messenger RNA production in human corneal endothelial cells. Invest Ophthalmol Vis Sci 1991;32:2747–2756.

10. Kawashima H, Gregerson DS. Corneal endothelial cells block T cell proliferation, but not T cell activation or responsiveness to exogenous IL-2. Curr Eye Res 1994;13:575–585.

11. Donnelly JJ, Zi MS, Rockey JH. A soluble product of human corneal fibroblasts inhibits lymphocyte activation. Enhancement by interferon-gamma. Exp Eye Res 1993;56:157–165.

12. Shams NB, Huggins EM Jr, Sigel MM. Regulation of mitogen-driven lymphoreticular cell activation by human corneal cells and interleukin-1. Cornea 1993;12:46–53.

13. Bouchard CS. The Ocular Immune Response. In JH Krachmer, MI Mannis, EJ Hollands (eds), Cornea: Fundamentals of Cornea and External Disease. St. Louis: Mosby, 1997;101.

14. Donnelly JJ, Chan LS, Xi MS, Rockey JH. Effect of human corneal fibroblasts on lymphocyte proliferation in vitro. Exp Eye Res 1988;47:61–70.

15. Cubitt CL, Lausch RN, Oakes JE. Differences in interleukin-6 gene expression between cultured human corneal epithelial cells and keratocytes. Invest Ophthalmol Vis Sci 1995;36:330–336.

16. Elner VM, Strieter RM, Pavilack MA, et al. Human corneal inerleukin-8: IL-1 and TNF-induced gene expression and secretion. Am J Ophthalmol 1991; 139:977–988.

17. Elner VM, Elner SG, Pavilack MA, et al. Rapid communication: intercellular adhesion molecule-1 in human corneal endothelium. Modulation and function. Am J Pathol 1991;138:525–536.

18. Foets BJ, van den Oord JJ, Volpes R, Missotten L. In situ immunohistochemical analysis of cell adhesion molecules on human corneal endothelial cells. Br J Ophthalmol 1992;76:205–209.

19. Seto SK, Gillette TE, Chandler JW. HLA-DR+/T6- Langerhans' cells of the human cornea. Invest Ophthalmol Vis Sci 1987;28:1719–1722.

20. Streilein JW, Toews GB, Bergstresser PR. Corneal allografts fail to express Ia antigens. Nature 1979;282:326–327.

21. Niederkorn JY, Peeler JS, Mellon J. Phagocytosis of particulate antigens by corneal epithelial cells stimulates interleukin-1 secretion and migration of Langerhans' cells into the central cornea. Reg Immunol 1989;2:83–90.

22. Asbell PA, Skittone LS, Epstein SP. Evaluation of chemotaxis by various cytokines of Ia+ Langerhans' cells into the corneas of C3H/HeJ mice. Invest Ophthalmol Vis Sci 1994;35(suppl):1293.

23. Roussel TJ, Osato MS, Wilhemus KR. Corneal Langerhans' cells migration following ocular contact sensitivity. Cornea 1983;2:27–30.

24. Streilein JW, Bradley D, Sano Y, Sonoda Y. Immunosuppressive properties of tissues obtained from eyes with experimentally manipulated corneas. Invest Ophthalmol Vis Sci 1996;37:413–424.

25. Iwata M, Yagihashi A, Roat MI, et al. Human leukocyte antigen-class II–positive human corneal epithelial cells activate allogeneic T cells. Invest Ophthalmol Vis Sci 1994;35:3991–4000.

26. McNeill JI. Indications and Outcomes. In JH Krachmer, MJ Mannis, EL Holland (eds), Cornea: Surgery of the Cornea and Conjunctiva. St. Louis: Mosby, 1997;1551.

27. Whitson WE, Weisenthal RW, Krachmer JH. Penetrating Keratoplasty. In W Tasman, EA Jaeger (eds), Duane's Ophthalmology. New York: Lippincott–Raven, 1996;1–28.

28. Aiello LP, Javitt JC, Canner JK. National outcomes of penetrating keratoplasty: risks of endophthalmitis and retinal detachment. Arch Ophthalmol 1993;111:509–513.

29. Thiel H-J. Signs and Symptoms of Corneal Graft Rejection. In M Zierhut, U Pleyer, H-J Thiel (eds), Immunology of Corneal Transplantation. Boston: Butterworth–Heinemann, 1994;140.

30. Seamone CD, Jackson WB. Immunology of the External Eye. Immunologic Considerations in Selected Ocular Diseases. In W Tasman, EA Jaeger (eds), Duane's Ophthalmology. New York: Lippincott–Raven, 1997;1–46.

31. Wackenheim-Urlacher A, Kantelip B, Falkenrodt A, et al. T-cell repertoire of normal, rejected, and pathological corneas: phenotype and function. Cornea 1995;14:450–456.

32. Nishi M, Matsubara M, Sugawara I, et al. An Immunohistochemical Study of Rejection Process in a Rat Penetrating Keratoplasty Model. In M Usui, S Ohno, S Aoki (eds), Ocular Immunology Today. Amsterdam: Elsevier, 1990; 99–102.

33. Otsuka H, Muramatsu R, Usui M. Immunohistochemical Study of Corneal Graft Rejection in Inbred Rats. In M Usui, S Ohno, S Aoki (eds), Ocular Immunology Today. Amsterdam: Elsevier, 1990;147–151.

34. He YG, Ross J, Niederkorn JY. Promotion of murine orthotopic corneal allograft survival by systemic administration of anti-CD4 monoclonal antibody. Invest Ophthalmol Vis Sci 1991;32:2723–2728.

35. Ayliffe W, Alam Y, Bell EB, et al. Prolongation of rat corneal graft survival by treatment with anti-CD4 monoclonal antibody. Br J Ophthalmol 1992;76:602–606.

36. Peeler J, Niederkorn JY, Matoba A. Corneal allografts induce cytotoxic T cell but not delayed hypersensitivity responses in mice. Invest Ophthalmol Vis Sci 1985;26:1516–1523.

37. Matsuda A, Tagawa Y, Matsuda H, Nishihira J. Identification and immunohistochemical localization of macrophage migration inhibitory factor in human cornea. FEBS Lett 1996;385:225–228.

38. Sher NA, Doughman DJ, Mindrup E, Minaai LA. Macrophage migration inhibition factor activity in the aqueous humor during experimental corneal xenograft and allograft rejection. Am J Ophthalmol 1976;82:858–865.

39. Torres PF, De Vos AF, van der Gaag R, et al. Cytokine mRNA expression during experimental corneal allograft rejection. Exp Eye Res 1996;63: 453–461.

40. Guymer RH, Mandel TE. A comparison of corneal, pancreas, and skin grafts in mice. A study of the determinants of tissue immunogenicity. Transplantation 1994;57:1251–1262.

41. Foster CS, Wu H, Merchant A. Systemic (serum) soluble interleukin-2 receptor levels in corneal transplant recipients. Documenta Ophthalmologica 1993;83:83–89.

42. Hoffmann F, Kruse HA, Meinhold H, et al. Interleukin-2 receptor–targeted therapy by monoclonal antibodies in the rat corneal graft. Cornea 1994; 13:440–446.

43. Herbort CP, de Smet MD, Roberge FG, et al. Treatment of corneal allograft rejection with the cytotoxin IL-2-PE40. Transplantation 1991;52:470–474.

44. Whitcup SM, Nussenblatt RB, Price FW Jr, Chan C-C. Expression of cell adhesion molecules in corneal graft failure. Cornea 1993;12:475–480.

45. Philipp W, Gottinger W. Leukocyte adhesion molecules in chronic inflammatory diseases of the cornea. Ophthalmologica 1993;207:19–29.

46. He Y, Mellon J, Apte R, Niederkorn JY. Effect of LFA-1 and ICAM-1 antibody treatment on murine corneal allograft survival. Invest Ophthalmol Vis Sci 1994;35:3218–3225.

47. Yamagami S, Obata H, Tsuru T, Isobe M. Suppression of corneal allograft rejection after penetrating keratoplasty by antibodies to ICAM-1 and LFA-1 in mice. Transplant Proc 1995;27:1899–1900.

48. Hori J, Yamagami S, Obata H, et al. Effect of monoclonal antibody to VLA-4 on corneal allograft survival in mice. Transplant Proc 1996;28:1990–1991.

49. Hutchinson IV, Alam Y, Ayliffe WR. The humoral response to an allograft. Eye 1995;9(pt 2):155–160.

50. Jager MJ, Vos A, Pasmans S, et al. Circulating cornea-specific antibodies in corneal disease and cornea transplantation. Graefes Arch Clin Exp Ophthalmol 1994;232:82–86.

51. Sanfilippo F, MacQueen JM, Vaughn WK, Foulks GN. Reduced graft rejection with good HLA-A and B matching in high-risk corneal transplantation. N Engl J Med 1986;315:29–35.

52. Boisjoly HM, Roy R, Dube I, et al. HLA-A,B and DR matching in corneal transplantation. Ophthalmology 1986;93:1290–1297.

53. The Collaborative Corneal Transplantation Studies Research Group. The Collaborative Corneal Transplantation Studies (CCTS). Effectiveness of histocompatibility matching in high-risk corneal transplantation. Arch Ophthalmol 1992;110:1392–1403.

54. Sonoda Y, Sano Y, Ksander B, Streilein JW. Characterization of cell-mediated immune responses elicited by orthotopic corneal allografts in mice. Invest Ophthalmol Vis Sci 1995;36:427–434.

55. Sano Y, Ksander BR, Streilein JW. Murine orthotopic corneal transplantation in high-risk eyes. Rejection is dictated primarily by weak rather than strong alloantigens. Invest Ophthalmol Vis Sci 1997;38:1130–1138.

56. Borderie VM, Lopez M, Vedie F, Laroche L. ABO antigen blood-group compatibility in corneal transplantation. Cornea 1997;16:1–6.

57. Rubsamen PE, McCulley J, Bergstresser PR, Streilein JW. On the Ia immunogenicity of mouse corneal allografts infiltrated with Langerhans' cells. Invest Ophthalmol Vis Sci 1984;25:513–518.

58. Gillette TE, Chandler JW, Greiner JV. Langerhans' cells of the ocular surface. Ophthalmology 1982;89:700–711.

59. Dana MR, Streilein JW. Loss and restoration of immune privilege in eyes with corneal neovascularization. Invest Ophthalmol Vis Sci 1996;37:2485–2494.

60. Hill JC, Sarvan J, Maske R, Els WJ. Evidence that UV-B irradiation decreases corneal Langerhans' cells and improves corneal graft survival in the rabbit. Transplantation 1994;57:1281–1284.

61. Sonoda Y, Streilein JW. Impaired cell-mediated immunity in mice bearing healthy orthotopic corneal allografts. J Immunol 1993;150:1727–1734.

62. Geiger K, Sarvetnick N. Local production of IFN-γ abrogates the intraocular immune privilege in transgenic mice and prevents the induction of ACAID. J Immunol 1994;153:5239–5246.

63. Sano Y, Okamoto S, Streilein JW. Induction of donor-specific ACAID can prolong orthotopic corneal allograft survival in "high-risk" eyes. Curr Eye Res 1997;16:1171–1174.

64. She SC, Steahly LP, Moticka EJ. Intracameral injection of allogeneic lymphocytes enhances corneal graft survival. Invest Ophthalmol Vis Sci 1990; 31:1950–1956.

65. She SC, Moticka EJ. Ability of intracamerally inoculated B and T cell enriched allogeneic lymphocytes to enhance corneal allograft survival. Int Ophthalmol 1993;17:1–7.

66. Yao Y-F, Inoue Y, Miyazaki D, et al. Correlation of anterior chamber-associated immune deviation with suppression of corneal epithelial rejection in mice. Invest Ophthalmol Vis Sci 1997;38:292–300.

67. Niederkorn JY, Mellon J. Anterior chamber-associated immune deviation promotes corneal allograft survival. Invest Ophthalmol Vis Sci 1996;37:2700–2707.

68. Hill JC. Immunosuppression in corneal transplantation. Eye 1995;9(pt 2):247–253.

69. Yamada J, Streilein JW. Induction of anterior chamber-associated immune deviation by corneal allografts placed in the anterior chamber. Invest Ophthalmol Vis Sci 1997;38:2833–2843.

70. Volker-Dieben HJ, D'Amaro J, Van Slooten H, Kruit PJ. The Effect of Cyclosporin A on Corneal Graft Survival. In M Zierhut, U Pleyer, H-U Thiel (eds), Immunology of Corneal Transplantation. Boston: Butterworth–Heinemann, 1994;239.

71. Hill JC. The use of cyclosporine in high-risk keratoplasty. Am J Ophthalmol 1989;107:506–510.

72. Miller K, Huber C, Niederwieser D, Gottinger W. Successful engraftment of high-risk corneal allografts with short-term immunosuppression with cyclosporine. Transplantation 1988;45:651–653.

73. Hill JC. Systemic cyclosporine in high-risk keratoplasty: long-term results. Eye 1995;9(pt 4):422–428.

74. Hoffmann F. Topical Cyclosporin A in Corneal Transplantation. In M Zierhut, U Pleyer, H-U Thiel (eds), Immunology of Corneal Transplantation. Boston: Butterworth–Heinemann, 1994;253.

75. Belin MW, Bouchard CS, Frantz S, Chmielinska J. Topical cyclosporine in high-risk corneal transplants. Ophthalmology 1989;96:1144–1150.

76. Maske R, Hill J, Horak S. Mixed lymphocyte culture responses in rabbits undergoing corneal grafting and topical cyclosporine treatment. Cornea 1994;13:324–330.

77. Nishi M, Herbort CP, Matsubara M, et al. Effects of the immunosuppressant FK506 on a penetrating keratoplasty rejection model in the rat. Invest Ophthalmol Vis Sci 1993;34:2477–2486.

78. Mills RA, Jones DB, Winkler CR, et al. Topical FK-506 prevents experimental corneal allograft rejection. Cornea 1995;14:157–160.

79. Hikita N, Lopez JS, Chan C-C, et al. Use of topical FK506 in a corneal graft rejection model in Lewis rats. Invest Ophthalmol Vis Sci 1997;38:901–909.

80. Benelli U, Lepri A, Del Tacca M, Nardi M. FK-506 delays corneal graft rejection in a model of corneal xenotransplantation. J Ocul Pharmacol Ther 1996;12:425–431.

81. Eastlund T. Infectious disease transmission through cell, tissue, and organ transplantation: reducing the risk through donor selection. Cell Transpl 1995;4:455–477.

82. Caron MJ, Wilson R. Review of the risk of HIV infection through corneal transplantation in the United States. J Am Optom Assoc 1994;65:173–178.

83. Hoft RH, Pflugfelder SC, Forster RK, et al. Clinical evidence for hepatitis B transmission resulting from corneal transplantation. Cornea 1997;16:132–137.

84. Sugar J, Mannis M. Grafting and the risk of hepatitis transmission: Is there reason to be cautious? Are we cautious enough? Cornea 1997;16:123–124.

85. Ross JR, Howell DN, Sanfilippo FP. Characteristics of corneal xenograft rejection in a discordant species combination. Invest Ophthalmol Vis Sci 1993;34:2469–2476.

86. Larkin DFP, Takano T, Standfield SD, Williams KA. Experimental orthotopic corneal xenotransplantation in the rat. Mechanisms of graft rejection. Transplantation 1995;60:491–497.

87. Larkin DFP, Williams KA. The host response in experimental corneal xenotransplantation. Eye 1995;9(pt 2):254–260.

Index